Con

Contents

Call for Ideas

Submit ideas for new cards in future editions of the *Peripheral Brain*.
Send your ideas to aphabooks@aphanet.org. Thanks!

Please let us know the most useful content or additional areas that
you'd like to see in the future to further increase the value of this product.

2018-19 Peripheral Brain for the PHARMACIST

Edited by
Jeanine P. Abrons, PharmD, MS

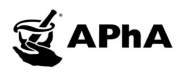

Washington, D.C.

Acquiring Editor: Janan Sarwar
Managing Editor: Jim Angelo
Editor: Ryan J. Quick
Cover Design, Layout, and Graphics: APhA Integrated Design and
Production Center

Published by the American Pharmacists Association,
2215 Constitution Avenue, NW, Washington, DC 20037-2985
www.pharmacist.com • www.pharmacylibrary.com

To comment on this product by e-mail, send your message to the publisher
at *aphabooks@aphanet.org*.

How to Order This Product
Online: www.pharmacist.com/shop
By phone: 800-878-0729 (770-250-0085 from outside the
U.S. and Canada)
VISA®, MasterCard®, and American Express® cards accepted.

Contributors

AUTHORS

JEANINE P. ABRONS, PharmD, MS
Clinical Assistant Professor/Director of
Student Pharmacists International Activities
University of Iowa College of Pharmacy
Iowa City, Iowa

ELISHA ANDREAS, PharmD
Pharmacist
Hartig Drug
Iowa City, Iowa

JENNA BLUNT
Postgraduate Year 1 Resident
John Hopkins Medicine
Baltimore, Maryland

MARK BOTTI, PharmD
Pharmacist
Albany Medical Center
Albany, New York

SARA E. DUGAN, PharmD, BCPP, BCPS
Associate Professor of Pharmacy Practice
Northeast Ohio Medical University
 College of Pharmacy
Rootstown, Ohio

BRITTANY HAYES, BS, RRT, RCP, PharmD
Post Graduate Year 1 Resident
Veterans Affairs Medical Center-
Tennessee Valley Healthcare System
Nashville, Tennessee

APRYL JACOBS, PharmD
Pharmacist
St. Peter's Hospital
Albany, New York

BEN LOMAESTRO, PharmD
Senior Clinical Pharmacy Specialist–
 Infectious Disease
Albany Medical Center
Albany, New York

ANH LUONG, PharmD Candidate 2018
University of Iowa College of Pharmacy
Iowa City, Iowa

ERICA MACEIRA, PharmD, BCPS, CACP
Clinical Pharmacy Specialist
Transplant and Anticoagulation
Albany Medical Center
Albany, New York

JASMINE MANGRUM
PharmD Candidate 2019
University of Iowa College of Pharmacy
Iowa City, Iowa

REBECCA PETRIK, PharmD
Pharmacist
Wheat Ridge, Colorado

MOLLY POLZIN, PharmD
Postgraduate Year 2 Resident
University of Nebraska Medical Center
Omaha, Nebraska

JESSICA RAMICH, PharmD
Clinical Pharmacy Specialist
Guthrie Corning Hospital
Big Flats, New York

ADRIENNE ROUILLER, PharmD
Clinical Pharmacist
Health Alliance Hospital
Leominster, Massachusetts

JOANNA RUSCH
PharmD Candiate 2018
University of Iowa, College of Pharmacy
Iowa City, Iowa

BREANNA SUNDERMAN, PharmD
Pharmacy Manager, CVS
Overland Park, Kansas

BRYAN PINCKNEY WHITE, PharmD
Infectious Diseases Clinical Pharmacist
Oklahoma University Medical Center
Oklahoma City, OKlahoma

ANGELA WOJTCZAK
PharmD Candidate 2018
University of Iowa, College of Pharmacy
Iowa City, Iowa

Acknowledgments

The editor and publisher gratefully acknowledge Jennifer Cerulli, PharmD, BCPS, and Renée Ahrens Thomas, PharmD, MBA, for their help in selecting the contents of previous editions; and Jennifer L. Adams, PharmD, EdD, and Keith D. Marciniak, BSPharm, who developed the concept of reference cards in an APhA resource that preceded *Peripheral Brain for the Pharmacist*. The editor and publisher gratefully recognize Alecia Heh for her involvement in previous versions of Diabetes related pages, and Eric P. Boateng for his work on the Medications with Adverse Withdrawal Effects from Abrupt Discontinuation pages.

A special thanks to Jing Wu, PharmD, MPH, for her efforts in reviewing this book. We would also like to thank the following PharmD Candidates: Meryam Gharbi, Olivia Johnson, Mark Sundh, Tina Nguyen, and Sonya Park. We additionally thank Michelle Powell for her time redesigning the layout of this edition.

Hypertension Management

High Blood Pressure Guideline Summary: The 2017 Guideline for the Prevention, Detection, Evaluation, & Management of High Blood Pressure in Adults represents an update of the Joint National Committee (JNC) guidelines from 2003. The guidelines include information from studies on related risk of CVD#, monitoring, & includes thresholds to start drug treatment & goals.

Classifying High Blood Pressure (BP) in Adults:

CATEGORY	SYSTOLIC Blood Pressure (SBP) in mm Hg		DIASTOLIC Blood Pressure (DBP) in mm Hg
Normal	< 120	AND	< 80
Elevated	120-129	AND	< 80
Hypertension (HTN)			
• Stage 1	130-139	OR	80-89
• Stage 2	≥ 140	OR	≥ 90

Patient with high SBP & DBP in 2 categories: select the higher category.
Caution: BP is based on an average of ≥ 2 readings taken on ≥ 2 occasions.
BP measurements in clinical trial may not represent typical level of care & patient motivation.

Use of CVD Risk Estimation* & Blood Pressure Threshold to Guide Drug Treatment

Use of BP-lowering medications are recommended for:

• ***Primary prevention*** of CVD# for patients with no history of CVD **AND** 10-year ASCVD^ risk < 10% & SBP ≥ 140 mm Hg or DBP ≥ 90 mm Hg
• ***Primary prevention*** of CVD for patients with 10-year ASCVD risk ≥ 10% & average SBP ≥ 130 mm Hg or average DBP ≥ 80 mm Hg
• ***Secondary prevention*** of recurrent CVD events for patients with clinical CVD & average SBP ≥ 130 mm Hg or average DBP ≥ 80 mm Hg

Initial Monotherapy Versus Initial Combination Drug Therapy

• ***Stage 1 hypertension (HTN) & BP goal < 130/80 mm Hg.***
Start one antihypertensive drug. Titrate dose & sequentially add other agents to achieve BP target.
• ***Stage 2 hypertension & average BP > 20/10 mm Hg above target.***
Start 2 first-line agents of different classes, either as separate agents or in fixed-dose combination.

Initial Medication Options

• ***First-line agents:*** ACE† inhibitors or ARBsΔ, thiazide diuretics, & CCBs▶

*ACC/AHA Pooled Cohort Equations: (http://tools.acc.org/ASCVD-Risk-Estimator/).
#: cardiovascular disease, ^: atherosclerotic cardiovascular disease
ASCVD was defined as a first Congenital Heart Disease death, non-fatal Myocardial Infarction or fatal or non-fatal stroke.
†ACE = Angiotensin conversion enzyme inhibitor; ΔARB = Angiotensin receptor blocker;
▶CCB = Calcium Channel Blockers

Considerations in Care – Management of High Blood Pressure

CONSIDERATION	DESCRIPTION	
Blood Pressure Management	• Accurate management is critical. • Consider out-of-office & self-monitoring to confirm & titrate medications. • Measurement values may vary depending on time & location taken.	
Screen/Manage Other CVD Risk Factors	• Smoking; diabetes; dyslipidemia; weight; low fitness; poor diet; stress; sleep apnea • Testing:	
	BASIC testing	Complete blood count; Fasting blood glucose; Lipid profile; Serum creatinine with estimated glomerular filtration rate (eGFR); Serum electrolytes (K^+; Na^{2+}; Ca^{2+}); Thyroid-stimulating hormone (TSH); Urinalysis; Electrocardiogram
	OPTIONAL testing	Echocardiogram; Uric acid; Urine albumin to creatinine ratio
Screen for Secondary Causes of HTN	• Screen for common secondary causes with new-onset or uncontrolled hypertension. • If more specific clinical symptoms are present, consider uncommon secondary causes. **What to Screen For**	
	COMMON Causes **Screen for secondary causes of hypertension‡** Primary aldosteronism (elevated aldosterone/renin ratio) CKD (eGFR < 60 mL/min/1.73 m²) Renal artery stenosis (young female, known atherosclerotic disease, worsening kidney function) Pheochromocytoma (episodic hypertension, palpitations, diaphoresis, headache) Obstructive sleep apnea (snoring, witnessed apnea, excessive daytime sleepiness)	• Abrupt onset • Age < 30 • Drug resistant/induced: uncontrolled BP after treatment with greater than or equal to 3 antihypertensives • Excessive target organ damage (e.g. cerebral vascular disease; retinopathy; left ventricular hypertrophy, heart failure (HF) with preserved ejection fraction (EF) or with reserved EF; coronary artery disease (CAD); Chronic kidney disease (CKD); peripheral artery disease; albuminuria) • OR onset of diastolic HTN in older adults • OR unprovoked or excessive hypokalemia.
	UNCOMMON Causes **(< 1%)**	• Acromegaly • Aortic coarctation • Congenital adrenal hyperplasia • Mineralocorticoid excess syndrome (not primary aldosteronism) • Cushing's syndrome • Hypo/hyper thyroidism or primary hyperparathyroidism • Phenochromocytoma/paraganglioma

Follow-up	ADULT PATIENT GROUP	FREQUENCY OF FOLLOW-UP
	Low-Risk with Elevated BP or Stage 1 HTN with ASCVD risk < 10%	Repeat BP after 3 to 6 months of non-pharmacological therapy
	Stage 1 HTN & High ASCVD Risk (≥ 10% 10-year ASCVD risk)	Repeat BP after 1 month of non-pharmacologic & antihypertensive drug therapy
	Stage 2 HTN	Evaluate by primary care provider (PCP) within 1 month of diagnosis; Treat with combo of non-pharmacologic & 2 antihypertensive drugs from different classes; Repeat evaluation in 1 month
	Very High Average BP (Systolic ≥ 160 mmHg or Diastolic ≥ 100 mm Hg)	Evaluate promptly; Monitor carefully & adjust dose upward as needed
	Normal BP	Repeat BP evaluation annually

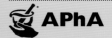

Hypertension Management (*continued*)

Causes of Drug Induced Elevations in Blood Pressure

Type of Medication	Medication	Recommendation
NON-PRESCRIPTION	**Alcohol**	• Limit to ≤ 1 drink [women]; ≤ 2 drinks [men];
	Caffeine	• Limit to < 300 mg/day. • Avoid use if hypertension is not controlled • May only have acute effect on BP
	Decongestants (Phenylephrine; Pseudoephedrine)	• Use for short duration. • Avoid in severe or uncontrolled HTN • Consider alternative.
	Herbals (Ephedra [Ma Huang]; St. John's Wort with MAOIs* and Yohimbine)	• Avoid use.
	Illicit Drug Use (Cocaine; Methamphetamine)	• Avoid use.
	Non-steroidal Anti-Inflammatory Agents (NSAIDs)	• Avoid use. • Consider alternative analgesic.
PRESCRIPTION	**Antidepressants** (MAOIs*; SNRIs;** TCAs***)	• Consider alternatives (Selective Seratonin Reuptake Inhibitors [SSRIs]). • Avoid tyramine containing foods if on MAOIs*
	Amphetamines (Amphetamine; methylphenidate; dexmethylphenidate; dextroamphetamine)	• Discontinue or decrease dose. • Consider alternatives (behavioral therapy).
	Atypical Antipsychotics (Clozapine; Olanzapine)	• Discontinue or limit use. • Consider alternatives (behavioral therapy; lifestyle modifications; other agents [with less weight gain, diabetes or dyslipidemia risk; e.g.: aripiprazole; ziprasidone).
	Oral Contraceptives	• Use low dose estrogens (20 to 30 mcg ethinyl estradiol) or progestin only. • Consider alternatives (e.g. barrier method; abstinence; intrauterine devices [IUD]). • Avoid if hypertension is not controlled.

*MAOI = Monoamine oxidase inhibitors; ** = SNRIs = Seratonin Norepinephrine Reuptake Inhibitors;
*** TCA = Tricyclic Antidepressants)

Hypertension Management *(continued)*

Management of High Blood Pressure in Specific Patient Populations

Population	Additional Description of Population	Target Blood Pressure (BP) or Recommended Treatment
Adults	Confirmed HTN* & known cardiovascular disease (CVD) or 10-year ASCVD** risk > 10%	< 130/80 mm Hg
	Confirmed HTN without added markers of ↑ CVD risk	< 130/80 mm Hg
Older Persons (>65 years old)	Non-institutionalized ambulatory community-dwelling adults with average systolic BP (SBP) ≥ 130 mm Hg	< 130 mm Hg
	HTN + high burden of comorbidity + limited life expectancy	Clinical judgment, patient preference, & team-based care; consider risk/benefit for decisions on intensity of BP ↓ & antihypertensive drugs
Hypertensive Adults + Heart Failure (HF) Risk	To prevent HF in hypertensive adults	< 130/80 mm Hg
Hypertension + HFrEF^	GDMT# (2) titrated to BP	< 130/80 mm Hg Non-dihydropyridine Calcium Channel Blockers [CCBs] not recommended
Hypertension + HFpEF^^	Volume overload	Control HTN with diuretics
	HFpEF & persistent HTN after volume overload is managed	Angiotensin Converting Enzyme Inhibitors (ACE (-)) or Angiotensin Receptor Blockers (ARBs) & beta blockers; Titrate to SBP < 130 mm Hg
Hypertension + CKD+	HTN + CKD	< 130/80 mm Hg
	HTN + CKD Stage ≥ 3 OR Stage 1 or 2 + albuminuria [≥ 300 mg/d, OR ≥ 300 mg/g albumin-to-creatinine ratio OR equivalent in 1st morning void]	ACE (-) to slow CKD progression or an ARB if ACE (-) intolerant
	HTN + CKD Stage ≥ 3 OR Stage 1 OR 2 + albuminuria [≥ 300 mg/d, OR ≥ 300 mg/g albumin-to-creatinine ratio OR equivalent in 1st morning void]	ARB if ACE(-) intolerant
Hypertension + DM##	BP ≥ 130/80 mm Hg	Start antihypertensive drug to goal of < 130/80 mm Hg; ACE (-), ARBs, diuretics, & CCBs = effective
	With albuminuria	ACE (-) or ARBs
Race & Ethnicity	Black adults with HTN but no HF or CKD, + DM	Thiazide-type diuretic or CCB for initial treatment
	Hypertensive adults, especially black adults	≥ 2 antihypertensives to achieve target of < 130/80 mm Hg

*: hypertension, **: Atherosclerotic cardiovascular disease, #: guideline-directed management & therapy, ^HFrEF: heart failure with reduced ejection fraction, ^^HFpEF: heart failure with preserved ejection fraction, + = CKD: chronic kidney disease, ##= diabetes mellitus

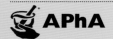

Atherosclerotic Cardiovascular Disease (ASCVD) Risk

Process of Evaluating a Patient Prior to Initiation of a Statin:

Initial evaluation prior to statin initiation:

- Fasting lipid panel
- ALT
- Creatinine Kinase (CK) [If indicated]
- Hemoglobin A1c [If diabetes status unknown]
- Consider evaluation for other secondary causes or conditions that may influence statin safety

Treat Laboratory Abnormalities

- Triglycerides $\geq$ 500 mg/dL
- LDL-C $\geq$ 190 mg/dL
- Unexplained ALT $\geq$ 3 x the Upper Limit of Normal (ULN)

Considerations:

Counsel all patients on lifestyle changes (e.g., nutrition and exercise) and evaluated for compliance.
To determine ASCVD risk for a patient, use the American Heart Association (AHA) and American College of Cardiology (ACC) online tool to calculate a patient's risk.
Apps also are available for many smart phones.
Drug-drug interactions with simvastatin may limit its use in certain patients. For patients on medications that interact with simvastatin, do not increase dose of simvastatin more than recommended when giving those medications concomitantly. When starting patients on simvastatin, doses > 40 mg should never be used due to risk of statin intolerance. Doses should not be increased to any dose > 40 mg for the same reason.
Switch from high-intensity to medium-intensity statin when drug-drug interactions, previous statin intolerance, or conditions that predispose patients to statin intolerance exist..
After initiation of statin, re-check fasting lipids within 4 to 12 weeks.
If change in lipids is as anticipated, monitor every 3-12 months, as appropriate.
If change in lipids is not as anticipated, re-enforce medication adherence and intensive lifestyle modifications and re-evaluate for secondary causes of dyslipidemia. After 4 to 12 weeks, re-evaluate and if patient is not at goal, consider increasing statins or adding on other lipid-lowering medications.
If patient has two consecutive fasting lipid panels with LDL-C < 40 mg/dL, consider decreasing dose.
Routine monitoring of creatinine kinase (CK) and hepatic function (Liver Function Tests: LFTs) is unnecessary unless patient is having symptoms of abnormal muscle pain or weakness for CK or hepatic dysfunction for LFTs.

Prepared by Mark Botti and Jeanine P. Abrons

Atherosclerotic Cardiovascular Disease (ASCVD) Risk

Process of Determining Intensity of Statin Therapy

Adults > 21 years and a candidate for statin therapy

| Clinical ASCVD | **Yes** | **High-intensity statin**
 Age ≤ 75 years
 Moderate intensity statin
 Age > 75 years OR
 If not a candidate for high-intensity |

No

| Low Density Lipoprotein (LDL-C) ≥ 190 mg/dL | **Yes** | **High-intensity statin**
 (Moderate-intensity statin if not candidate for high-intensity statin) |

No

| Diabetes Mellitus AND Age 40 to 75 AND LDL-C 70 to 189 mg/dL | **Yes** | **Moderate-intensity statin**
 Estimated 10-year ASCVD Risk ≥ 7.5%: High-intensity statin |

No

| LDL-C 70- to 189 mg/dL AND Age 40 to 75 AND 10-year ASCVD risk ≥ 7.5% | **Yes** | **Moderate- or high-intensity statin** |

All other patients: Determine all risk factors for ASCVD and discuss risks vs. benefits of statin therapy with other clinicians and patients.

Statin Intensities			
Intensity of Therapy	**High Intensity**	**Moderate Intensity**	**Low Intensity**
Impact to Low-Density Lipoproteins (LDLs)	LDL-C anticipated decrease of ≥50%	LDL-C anticipated decrease of 30 to 50%	LDL-C anticipated decrease of < 30%
Dosing of Medications	Atorvastatin dose of 40 to 80 mg	Atorvastatin dose of 10 to 20 mg	
		Fluvastatin dose of 40 mg BID	Fluvastatin dose of 20 to 40 mg
		Fluvastatin XL (Extended Release) 80 mg	
		Lovastatin dose of 40 mg	Lovastatin dose of 20 mg
		Pitavastatin dose of 2 to 4 mg	Pitavastatin dose of 1 mg
		Pravastatin dose of 40 to 80 mg	Pravastatin dose of 10 to 20 mg
	Rosuvastatin dose of 20 to 40 mg	Rosuvastatin dose of 5 to 10 mg	
		Simvastatin dose of 20 to 40 mg	Simvastatin dose of 10 mg

Prepared by Mark Botti and Jeanine P. Abrons

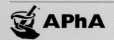

Information Required for Calculation of Atherosclerotic Cardiovascular Disease (ASCVD) Risk

Risk Factor	Potential Responses
Sex	• Male • Female
Age (in years)	• The risk calculation for adults ages 40 to 79 without clinical ASCVD & with LDL < 190 mg/dL
Race or Ethnicity	• African American • White • Other
Total Cholesterol	• Range from 130 to 320 mg/dL
Low Density Lipoprotein (LDL-C)	• Range from 30 to 300 mg/dL
High Density Lipoprotein (HDL-C)	• Range from 20 to 100 mg/dL
Systolic Blood Pressure	• Range from 90 to 200 mg/dL
High Blood Pressure Treatment	• Yes • No
Diagnosis of Diabetes	• Yes • No
Smoker	• Yes • No • Former

Additional Tools/Resources Available at: *http://tools.acc.org/ASCVD-Risk-Estimator-Plus/ (Accessed 2017)*

Prepared by Mark Botti

Associated Goals with Lipids

Age	No Known Risk Factors	ASCVD Risk Factor(s)*	ASCVD
< 40	No statin therapy	Moderate or high intensity statin dosing	High intensity statin dosing
40-75	Moderate intensity statin dosing	High intensity statin dosing	High intensity statin dosing
> 75[a]	Moderate intensity statin dosing	Moderate or high intensity statin dosing	High intensity statin dosing

a: If patient has change to Acute Coronary Syndrome (ACS) and LDL cholesterol > 50 mg/dL and cannot tolerate high dose statins, consider moderate intensity statin dosing plus the addition of ezetimibe.

*ASCVD risk factors include low density lipoprotein (LDL) ≥ 100 mg/dL, high blood pressure, smoking, overweight or obesity, and family history of premature ASCVD.

Note:
- *If a patient is not taking a statin, it is reasonable to obtain a lipid profile at diabetes diagnosis, or at an initial medical evaluation, or every 5 years, or more often if indicated. Refer to ASCVD risk card for further guidance on initiating statin therapy.*
- *Recommendations for statin therapy should be made in addition to lifestyle therapy.*

Prepared by Jeanine P. Abrons, Molly Polzin, and Elisha Andreas

Cholesterol Management:
Use of Drug Classes Other than Statins

Results other than high LDL-C:
Some patients with metabolic syndrome also may have low HDL-C or high triglycerides. The AHA/ACC guidelines for prevention of coronary artery disease recommend consideration of additional medications directed at these lipids such as niacin and fibrates.

When to Consider Use of Non-Statins:
May consider treatment with non-statin medications in high-risk patients with the following clinical scenarios:
• Less-than anticipated response to statins (after compliance has been confirmed)
• Inability to tolerate a less than recommended intensity of statin
• Complete intolerance to statin therapy

High-risk patients include:
• Patients with clinical ASCVD
• Primary elevations of LDL-C ≥ 190 mg/dL
• Patients with diabetes.

Fibrates and Omega-3 Fatty Acids may be considered in patients with persistent triglycerides > 500 mg/dL after lifestyle modification and treatment of causes

Drug Classes Other Than Statins		
Drug Class	Safety Considerations	Monitoring
Bile Acid Sequestrants	**Do not use if:** • Fasting triglycerides (TG) > 300 mg/dL • Type III Hyperlipoproteinemia **Use cautiously in patients with:** • Triglycerides (TG) 250 to 299 mg/dL **Discontinue use if:** • TG increase to > 400 mg/dL	• Baseline: fasting lipid profile • Re-evaluate 3 months after initiation and every 6 to 12 months thereafter
Cholesterol-Absorption Inhibitors	Discontinue with ALT (Alanine Aminotransferase) persistently > 3 times the Upper Limit of Normal (ULN)	• Baseline: ALT/AST (Aspartate Transaminase) • When taken concomitantly with statins, monitor as clinically indicated
Fibrates	Gemfibrozil should not be used in conjunction with statins due to increased risk of muscle toxicities Fenofibrate may be considered in conjunction with low- or moderate-intensity statins	• Renal function should be evaluated prior to initiation of fibrate, within 3 months of initiation, and every 6 months thereafter • Do not initiate, and discontinue if estimated glomerular filtration rate (eGFR) is persistently < 30 mL/min/1.73 m^2 • If eGFR is 30 to 59 mL/min/1.73 m^2, dose of fenofibrate should not be higher than 54 mg
Niacin	**Do not use if or with:** • ALT/AST ≥ 2 to 3 times ULN • Persistent, severe cutaneous reactions occur • Hyperglycemia • Acute gout • Gastrointestinal (GI) symptoms • New onset atrial fibrillation OR • Weight loss occurs • In patients who develop cutaneous reactions: refer to guidelines • Re-evaluate use in patients who develop other side effects • May consider niacin as adjunct for ↓ TG. Not for use with high dose statins and well-controlled LDL cholesterol	• Baseline: ALT/AST, fasting blood glucose or A1c, uric acid • Re-evaluate during titration and every 6 months once maintenance dose is determined
Omega-3 Fatty Acids	• Minimal safety considerations	• Evaluate for GI disturbances, skin changes, and bleeding

Prepared by Mark Botti

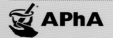

Direct Oral Anticoagulants

Medication/Consideration	Dabigatran (Pradaxa®) *Direct Thrombin Inhibitor (DTI)*	Rivaroxaban (Xarelto®) *Anti-Factor Xa Inhibitor*
FDA Approved Indications T = Treatment P = Prophylaxis	• Stroke/emboli prevention in non-valvular atrial fibrillation (NVAF)[T] • Deep vein thrombosis (DVT)/pulmonary embolism (PE) after 5 to 10 days of parenteral therapy[T] • ↓ DVT & PE recurrence in patients previously treated[P] • For DVT & PE prophylaxis in patients who have undergone hip replacement[P]	• Stroke/emboli prevention in NVAF[T] • DVT & PE[T] • DVT/PE risk ↓ after 6 months of prior treatment[P] • DVT/PE prophylaxis post hip/knee replacement[P]

Usual Dosage (T = Treatment, P = Prophylaxis)

Dabigatran:

Indication	T/P	Dose (Oral) – CrCl >30 mL/minute *After 5 to 10 days of parenteral therapy
NVAF	T	• 150 mg BID
DVT/PE*	T	• 150 mg BID
	P	• 150 mg BID after prior T
DVT/PE after hip replaced	P	• 110 mg on day 1, then 220 mg daily; start 1–4 hours after surgery/hemostasis achieved; for 28–35 days

Rivaroxaban:

Indication	T/P	Dose (Oral)
NVAF	T	• 20 mg daily
DVT/PE	T	• 15 mg BID x 21 days, then 20 mg daily
	P	• After 6 months of therapy: 10 mg daily per PI after prior T, with food
Post-Hip/Knee Prophylaxis	P	• Knee: 10 mg daily x 12 days • Hip: 10 mg daily x 35 days

Dose Adjustments (Based on Creatinine Clearance (CrCl))

Dabigatran:

Indication	T/P	Dose (Oral) – CrCl >30 mL/minute *After 5 to 10 days of parenteral therapy
NVAF	T	• At CrCl 15 to 30 mL/min: 75 mg BID • At CrCl <15 mL/min or dialysis: not recommended
DVT/PE*	T	• At ≤ 30 mL/min: avoid use
DVT/PE after hip replaced	P	• At CrCl ≤30 mL/min or on dialysis: Dosing recommendations cannot be provided

Rivaroxaban:

Indication	T/P	Dose (Oral)
NVAF	T	• At CrCl 15 to 50 mL/min: 15 mg daily • At CrCl <15mL/min: avoid use
Post-Hip/Knee Prophylaxis	T	• At CrCl <30 mL/min: avoid use
	P	• At CrCl 30-50 ml/min: monitor for bleeding • Start 6-10 hours after surgery if adequate hemostasis with rivaroxaban for post-hip/knee prophylaxis

Significant Drug Interactions	Dabigatran	Rivaroxaban
	• Serious interactions & dose adjustments required with P-gp inducers/inhibitors; ketoconazole; dronedarone - See package insert for complete list.	• Serious interactions & dose adjustments required with P-gp inducers/inhibitors; cytochrome P450 3A4 inducers/inhibitors - See package insert.
Miscellaneous Considerations	• Must administer capsule whole with full glass of water, do not break, chew, crush, or open • ESRD: Warfarin remains the drug of choice (DOC) per AHA/ACC • Cannot administer per tube	• Doses >10 mg MUST be taken with food; best with **evening meal if dosed once daily for NVAF** • ESRD: Warfarin remains the drug of choice (DOC) per AHA/ACC • Can be crushed

AHA = American Heart Association; ACC = American College of Cardiology

Direct Oral Anticoagulants *(continued)*

Medication/ Consideration	Apixaban (Eliquis®) *Anti-factor Xa Inhibitor*			Edoxaban (Savaysa®)		
FDA Approved Indications *T = Treatment* *P = Prophylaxis*	• Stroke/emboli prevention in non-valvular atrial fibrillation (NVAF)[T] • Deep vein thrombosis (DVT)/pulmonary embolism (PE)[T] • DVT/PE risk ↓ after prior T • For DVT & PE prophylaxis in patients who have undergone hip replacement[P]			• Stroke/emboli prevention in NVAF[T]: **Contraindicated in CrCl > 95 mL/min due to ↑ risk of ischemic stroke compared to warfarin** • Not recommended for CrC <15mL/min • DVT/PE Treatment after 5-10 days of parenteral anticoagulant[T]		
Usual Dosage *T = Treatment* *P = Prophylaxis* *^: Start 12 to 24 h after surgery*	**Indication**	**T/P**	**Dose (Oral)**	**Indication**	**T/P**	**Dose (Oral)** *^After 5 to 10 days of parenteral therapy*
	NVAF	T	• 5 mg BID	NVAF	T	• 60 mg daily **(Contraindicated with CrCL > 95 mL/min due to ↑ risk of ischemic stroke compared to warfarin)**
	DVT treatment	T P	• 10 mg BID for 7 days, then 5 mg BID • 2.5 mg BID after at least 6 months of T for DVT or PE	DVT/PE	T	• 60 mg daily • Patient weight ≤ 60 kg or with P-gp inhibitors or with short term use of macrolide antibiotics: 30 mg daily
	Post-Hip/Knee Prophylaxis	P	• For Knee Replacement: 2.5 mg BID for 12 days • For Hip Replacement: 2.5 mg BID for 35 days			
Dose Adjustments *^: in dialysis may use dosing; weak evidence* *Based on Creatinine Clearance (CrCl)*	**Indication**	**T/P**	**Dose (Oral)** *^Dose adjust in CrCl < 25 mL/min or SCR > 2.5 not studied*	**Indication**	**T/P**	**Dose (Oral)**
	NVAF	T	• If patient has any 2 traits: age ≥ 80; weight ≤ 60 kg; serum creatinine (SCr) ≥ 1.5 mg/dL: THEN 2.5 mg BID	NVAF	T	• At CrCl 15 to 50 mL/min: 15 mg daily
	DVT/PE; Post Knee/Hip Prophylaxis		• No dose adjustment for renal impairment for ESRD on dialysis; Use in CrCl < 15 mL/min not studied.	DVT/PE	T	• At 15 to 50 mL/min or ≤ 60 kg who use certain P-gp inhibitors: 30 mg daily
Significant Drug Interactions	• Serious interactions & dose adjustments required with dual use of P-gp inducers/inhibitors; dual use of cytochrome P450 3A4 inducers/inhibitors - See package insert for complete list.			• Serious interactions & dose adjustments required with P-gp inhibitor in T of NVAF, for DVT/PE, ENGAGE AF-TIMI 48: dose ↓ led to ↓ levels compared to full dose T, DVT/PE no dose ↓ with concomitant use - See package insert for complete list.		
Miscellaneous Considerations	• Can be taken with or without food • ESRD: Warfarin remains drug of choice (DOC) per AHA/ACC		• Can be crushed • ESRD/HD approval based on case reports and case series; Use caution & consider alternative	• Can be taken with or without food • No data on crushing &/or mixing/giving thru feeding tubes • ESRD: Warfarin remains the drug of choice (DOC) per AHA/ACC		

Prepared by Apryl Jacobs, Erica Maceira, and Jeanine P. Abrons

AHA = American Heart Association; ACC = American College of Cardiology

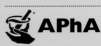 **APhA**

Injectable Anticoagulants

	Unfractionated Heparin	Enoxaparin (Lovenox®)	Dalteparin (Fragmin®)	Fondaparinux (Arixtra®)
Dosing				
Prophylaxis	• 5000 units SC every 8 hours or 5000 units SC every 12 hours	• 30 mg SC every 12 hours OR 40 mg SC every 24 hours • Creatinine Clearance (CrCl) < 30 mL/min: 30 mg SC every 24 hours • Do not use in dialysis	• 5000 units SC every 24 hours • May use 2500 units SC every 24 hours for low to moderate DVT risk in abdominal surgery • May use 2500 units SC 2 hours before surgery then 2500 units at least 4 to 8 hours after surgery (or later if hemostasis not achieved) then 5000 units SC every 24 hours • Do not use in dialysis	• 2.5 mg SC every 24 hours • Do not use in patients with CrCl < 30 mL/min or patients < 50 kg
VTE Treatment	• SC: 333 units/kg SC once followed by 250 units/kg SC every 12 hours • IV: 80 units/kg or 5000 units IV bolus then infusion of 18 units/kg (or 1000 units/hour) titrated to APTT or antifactor Xa assay (anti-Xa) • Goal: APTT = 1.5 to 2.5 x normal, Anti-Xa = 0.3–0.7	• 1 mg/kg SC every 12 hours OR • 1.5 mg/kg SC every 24 hours • CrCl < 30 mL/min: 1 mg/kg SC every 24 hours • Do not use in dialysis	• 100 units/kg SC every 12 hours OR • 200 units/kg SC every 24 hours • Do not use in patients with CrCl < 30 mL/min	• < 50 kg: 5 mg SC every 24 hours • 50 to 100 kg: 7.5 mg SC every 24 hours • > 100 kg: 10 mg SC every 24 hours • Do not use in patients with CrCl < 30 mL/min
Half-life	• 1 to 2 hours • Impacted by obesity; renal function; malignancy; and presence of pulmonary embolism	• 5 to 7 hours • Impacted by renal function	• 2 to 5 hours • Impacted by renal function	• 17 to 21 hours • Impacted by renal function
Excretion	• Primarily hepatic but also by reticuloendothelial system • Higher dose: renal elimination may play more of a role	• Excretion: renal (dose dependent)	• Excretion: primarily renal (dose dependent)	• Excretion: urine (77% excreted unchanged)
Inhibited Factors*	• Factors IIa, IXa, Xa, XIa, XIIa • Plasmin	• Factors Xa and IIa	• Factors Xa and IIa	• Factor Xa

*All act through antithrombin III (so in patients with antithrombin III deficiency these agents will predominantly be ineffective depending on the degree of deficiency); SC = Subcutaneous; IV = Intravenous

Injectable Anticoagulants *(continued)*

FDA Approved Indications

Indications (X = Indicated)	Enoxaparin	Dalteparin	Fondaparinux
Deep vein thrombosis (DVT) prophylaxis in abdominal surgery	X	X	X
DVT prophylaxis in knee replacement surgery	X	-------------------	X
DVT prophylaxis in hip replacement surgery	X	X	X (Hip fracture/replacement)
DVT prophylaxis in medical patients	X	X	-------------------
Inpatient treatment of acute DVT with or without pulmonary embolism (PE)	X	-------------------	X
Outpatient treatment of acute DVT without PE	X	-------------------	X
Prophylaxis for unstable angina and non-Q-wave MI	X	X	-------------------
Treatment of acute STEMI managed medically or with subsequent PCI	X	-------------------	-------------------
Treatment of acute PE	-------------------	-------------------	X (with warfarin when initial treatment is administered in the hospital)
Cancer patients with acute DVT and/or PE	-------------------	X	-------------------

Prepared by Erica Maceira and Apryl Jacobs

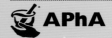

Perioperative Management of Direct Oral Anticoagulants

Medication/Half Life (T ½)	Renal Function (Creatinine Clearance [CrCl])	Low Bleeding Risk Surgery: Timing of Last Dose	High Bleeding Risk Surgery: Timing of Last Dose	When to Resume Therapy LOW Bleeding Risk Surgery	When to Resume Therapy HIGH Bleeding Risk Surgery
Dabigatran (Pradaxa®)					
T ½ = 12 to 17 hours; 14 to 17 hours in elderly	> 50 mL/min	2 days before procedure	3 days before procedure	Resume on the day after procedure (24 hours postoperative)	Resume 2 to 3 days after procedure (48 to 72 hours postoperative)
T ½ = 15 to 18 hours	30 to 50 mL/min	3 days before procedure	4 to 5 days before procedure		
Rivaroxaban (Xarelto®)					
T ½ = 5 to 9 hours	> 50 mL/min	2 days before procedure	3 days before procedure	Resume on the day after procedure (24 hours postoperative)	Resume 2 to 3 days after procedure (48 to 72 hours postoperative)
T ½ = 9 hours	30 to 50 mL/min	2 days before procedure	3 days before procedure		
T ½ = 9 to 10 hours	15 to 29 mL/min	Varies based on patient/procedure	Varies based on patient/procedure		
Apixaban (Eliquis®)					
T ½ = 12 hours	> 50 mL/min	2 days before procedure	3 days before procedure	Resume on the day after procedure (24 hours postoperative)	Resume 2 to 3 days after procedure (48 to 72 hours postoperative)
T ½ =	15 to 29 mL/min	Varies based on patient/procedure	Varies based on patient/procedure		
T ½ = 17 to 18 hours	30 to 50 mL/min	2 days before procedure	3 days before procedure		
Edoxaban (Savgaysa®)					
T ½ = 10 to 14 hours	> 50 mL/min	2 days before procedure	3 days before procedure	Resume on the day after procedure (24 hours postoperative)	Resume 2 to 3 days after procedure (48 to 72 hours postoperative)

NOTE: For patients at high risk for thromboembolism & bleed risk after surgery, consider administering a reduced dose of dabigatran (75 mg BID), rivaroxaban (10 mg daily), or apixaban (2.5 mg BID) on the evening after surgery and on the first postoperative day.

These recommendations are for patients not undergoing neuraxial procedures. For patients undergoing neuraxial procedures, see American Society of Regional Anesthesia and Pain Medicine guidelines: https://journals.lww.com/rapm/Fulltext/2015/05000/Interventional_Spine_and_Pain_Procedures_in.2.aspx.

Doherty J, Gluckman T, Hucker W, et al. 2017 ACC Expert Consensus Decision Pathway for Periprocedural Management of Anticoagulation in Patients With Nonvalvular Atrial Fibrillation: A Report of the American College of Cardiology Clinical Expert Consensus Document Task Force. *J Am Coll Cardiol.* 2017 Feb 21;69(7):871-898.

Prepared by Erica Maceria and Apryl Jacobs

Common Warfarin Drug Interactions

Drug Class or Medication That Interacts with Warfarin	Impact on Warfarin levels: Potential Management
Antibiotics E.g. Ciprofloxacin; Clarithromycin; Erythromycin; Metronidazole; Sulfamethoxazole /Trimethoprim	Majority ↑ ***Metronidazole:*** ↑; Consider alternatives. If used together, consider ↓ warfarin dose by 25 to 50% ***Dicloxacillin:*** ↓; more significant if course >14 days *Rifampin:* ↓; May consider ↑ of warfarin dose by 25-50%. *Ciprofloxacin:* ↑ At 2-5 days; May consider ↓ warfarin dose by 10-15% *Clarithromycin:* At 3-7 days; May ↓ dose warfarin by 15-25% *Erythromycin:* At 3-5 days; May consider ↓ warfarin dose by 10-15% *Sulfamethoxazole/Trimethoprim:* ↑ At 2-5 days; May consider ↓ warfarin dose by 25-40%
Antifungal Medications: E.g. Fluconazole; Miconazole	↑ At 2 to 3 days; Consider initial dose ↓ by 25-30%; May need to ↓ up to 80% with fluconazole
Antidepressants: E.g. Quetiapine; SSRIs; Tramadol	↑; *Tramadol:* Warfarin dose may need to be ↓ by 25-30%
Antiplatelet Medications	Does not increase INR, just ↑ bleeding risk. Monitor for signs/symptoms.
Anticoagulant Medications	Does not increase INR, just ↑ bleeding risk. Monitor for signs/symptoms.
Amiodarone	↑; Slow ↑ over time (e.g. 6 to 8 weeks); Empiric warfarin dose by 10-25% at week 1; may ↓ warfarin dose by 25-60% eventually
Acetaminophen	↑; With high doses (limited dose to <2,000 mg/day → Avoid use of higher doses if possible); Onset at 2-5 days
Carbamazepine	↓; Warfarin dose may need to be ↑ by 50-100%; ↓ warfarin dose by 50% when stopping
Fenofibrate	↑; Warfarin dose may need to be ↑ by 50-100%; ↓ warfarin dose by 50% when stopping
Gemfibrozil	↑; May ↓ dose warfarin by 10-15%
Phenobarbital	↓; Warfarin dose may need to be ↑ by 30-60%
Rosuvastatin	↑; May ↓ dose warfarin by 10-25%
Alternative Therapies *Note: Please refer to additional reference for more extensive list*	↑ Levels ↓ Levels C: Cannabis; Capsicum; Chamomile; Clove; Cranberry G: Ginseng; Green Tea; Goldenseal G: Garlic; Ginger; Gingko; Grapefruit Other: Noni; Parsley; St. John's Wort; Yarrow

For all significant drug interactions, monitor INR more often. Note: This table is not all inclusive; It provides a guidance for recall of common interactions that require dose adjustment of warfarin; Eg. Anti-inflammatory & anti-platelet medications should have increased monitoring for signs & symptoms of bleeding; SSRI = Selective Serotonin Reuptake Inhibitor;

Sample References: http://www.ncbi.nlm.nih/pmc/articles/PMC1942100/pdf/200708146s0018p369.pdf (Accessed 2017); Alternative Therapies Reference: National Center for Complementary and Alternative Medicine (http://nccam.nih.gov/health/herbsataglance.html (Accessed 2017)

Prepared by Jeanine P. Abrons and Erica Maceira

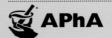

Warfarin Dosing According to the 9th Edition of CHEST Guidelines

Monitoring Based on CHEST Guidelines

- In hospitalized patients, INR monitoring is typically performed daily until therapeutic range is achieved and maintained for at least 2 consecutive days.
- In an outpatient setting, INRs will be monitored more frequently initially (e.g., every 1 to 3 days) and then frequency between INRs can be increased once a stable dose is achieved.
- For outpatient with consistently stable INRs, testing frequency may be extended up to 12 weeks (rather than every 4 weeks).
- Optimal frequency of monitoring may be impacted by patient compliance, co-morbid conditions, medication use, and dose response.
- It is important to know the reason for being on warfarin as this will impact the duration of therapy.

Consider influence of factors which may be associated with higher risk of bleeding:

- Advanced age
- Serious co-morbid conditions (cancer; renal insufficiency; liver disease; arterial hypertension; prior stroke; alcohol abuse; other therapies)

If fluctuations occur—consider the reasons for the fluctuation:

- Inaccuracy of INR testing
- Changes in dietary Vitamin K intake
- Changes in absorption/distribution/metabolism/excretion of Vitamin K or warfarin

Management of Out of Range INRs Based on CHEST Guidelines

- For previously stable patients with a single out-of-range INR of ≤ 0.5 below or above the therapeutic range, the current dose may be continued and testing can be done within 1 to 2 weeks.
  - Risk to patient is considered to be low.
- For stable patients with single sub-therapeutic INR, do not routinely bridge with a parenteral anticoagulant.
- With major bleeding, rapid reversal of anticoagulation with four-factor Prothrombin complex concentrate is suggested rather than with plasma.
- Add Vitamin K 5 to 10 mg administered by slow IV injection rather than reversal with coagulation factors alone.

Sample INR Level and Corresponding Evidence of Bleeding:

INR Level and Evidence of Bleeding	Recommendation
4.5 to 10 and No Evidence of Bleeding	Routine use of Vitamin K not recommended
Greater than 10 and No Evidence of Bleeding	Administer oral Vitamin K
Evidence of Bleeding	Kcentra and Vitamin K

Warfarin Dosing According to the 9th Edition
of CHEST Guidelines *(continued)*

Target INRs
- The CHEST 9th Edition Guidelines recommend therapeutic INRs of 2 to 3 rather than lower (< 2) or higher (3 to 5) ranges (Grade 1B).
- Higher intensity INR ranges exist for patients with mechanical mitral valves or with mechanical aortic valve & other risk factors.

Initiation of Warfarin Dosing Based on CHEST Guidelines
- CHEST 9th Edition Guidelines suggest patients sufficiently healthy to be treated as outpatients may start at 10 mg for 2 days followed by dosing based on INR.
- In patients with acute thromboembolism, therapy may be started on day 1 or 2 of an injectable anticoagulant rather than waiting to start.
- Many patients will be started at doses between 5 and 10 mg.
- Examples of when to consider a starting dose of < 5 mg:

• Elderly	• Impaired nutrition
• Liver disease	• High bleeding risk
• Congestive heart failure	

- 2 to 3 mg initial dose appropriate for patient with heart valve replacement.

Counseling Points Related to Warfarin
- Many drug interactions exist. Instruct the patient about the likelihood of a drug interaction and to report all medication changes.
- Know the reason that warfarin is being prescribed, as this will impact the duration of therapy.

Consistency is key with

• Medication compliance	• INR monitoring
• Medication interactions	• Vitamin K intake

Ask questions if recent changes have occurred:

• Does the new med interact?	• Recent illness?
• Dietary changes?	• How does patient take medication (assess compliance)?

Signs & symptoms of bleeding:
- Stress the importance of reporting signs or symptoms to the doctor & pharmacist.
- This may mean that warfarin is dosed at too high of a level.

Warfarin Strengths & Colors

1 mg:	2 mg:	2.5 mg:	3 mg:	4 mg:	5 mg:	6 mg:	7.5 mg:	10 mg:
Pink	Purple	Green	Brown	Blue	Orange	Teal	Yellow	White

Other Warfarin Resources (accessed November 2017)
- http://www.warfarindosing.org/source/home.aspx
- http://www.coumadin.bmscustomerconnect.com

Prepared by Jeanine P. Abrons

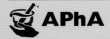

Alterations to Warfarin Dose Maintenance Therapy

This flow chart does not replace the need for clinical decision making. Decisions regarding patient care should be made in accordance with clinical judgment. Care should be given as medically necessary in the patient's best interest based upon independent clinical reasoning, clinician judgment, and objective data. Percentage adjustments may vary by institutional nomogram as well (e.g., INR < 2, increase by 10 to 15%; INR 3.1 to 3.5, decrease by 0 to 10%). This card was created by referencing multiple nomograms.

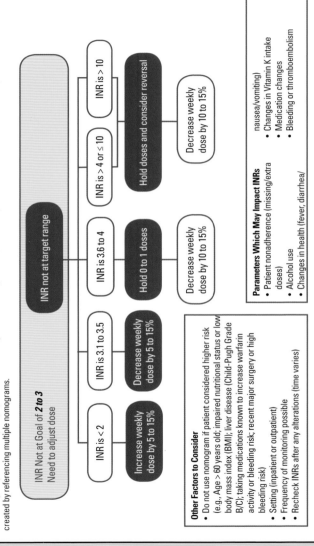

Other Factors to Consider
- Do not use nomogram if patient considered higher risk (e.g., Age > 60 years old; impaired nutritional status or low body mass index (BMI); liver disease (Child-Pugh Grade B/C); taking medications known to increase warfarin activity or bleeding risk; recent major surgery or high bleeding risk)
- Setting (inpatient or outpatient)
- Frequency of monitoring possible
- Recheck INRs after any alterations (time varies)

Parameters Which May Impact INRs
- Patient nonadherence (missing/extra doses)
- Alcohol use
- Changes in health (fever, diarrhea/nausea/vomiting)
- Changes in Vitamin K intake
- Medication changes
- Bleeding or thromboembolism

INR Not at Goal of **2 to 3**
Need to adjust dose

INR is < 2 → Increase weekly dose by 5 to 15%

INR is 3.1 to 3.5 → Decrease weekly dose by 5 to 15%

INR not at target range

INR is 3.6 to 4 → Hold 0 to 1 doses → Decrease weekly dose by 10 to 15%

INR is > 4 or ≤ 10

INR is > 10

Hold doses and consider reversal → Decrease weekly dose by 10 to 15%

Alterations to Warfarin Dose Maintenance Therapy *(continued)*

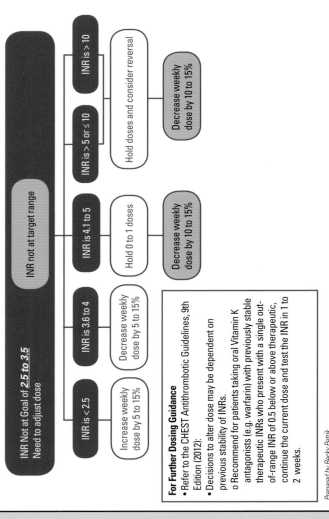

INR Not at Goal of _2.5 to 3.5_
Need to adjust dose

INR not at target range

INR is < 2.5	INR is 3.6 to 4	INR is 4.1 to 5	INR is > 5 or ≤ 10	INR is > 10

Increase weekly dose by 5 to 15%

Decrease weekly dose by 5 to 15%

Hold 0 to 1 doses

Decrease weekly dose by 10 to 15%

Hold doses and consider reversal

Decrease weekly dose by 10 to 15%

For Further Dosing Guidance
- Refer to the CHEST Antithrombotic Guidelines, 9th Edition (2012):
- Decisions to alter dose may be dependent on previous stability of INRs.
  - o Recommend for patients taking oral Vitamin K antagonists (e.g. warfarin) with previously stable therapeutic INRs who present with a single out-of-range INR of 0.5 below or above therapeutic, continue the current dose and test the INR in 1 to 2 weeks.

Prepared by Becky Petrik

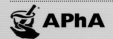

Diabetes Treatment Guidelines

For more comprehensive information about current approaches to the diagnosis and treatment of diabetes, visit the American Diabetes Association Standards of Medical Care—2018 Website at *https://professional.diabetes.org/content-page/standards-medical-care-diabetes (Accessed 2018).*

Criteria for Diagnosis of Diabetes

Diagnostic Tool	Value Associated with Diagnosis of Diabetes
Fasting Plasma Glucose (FPG)#	≥ 126 mg/dL • In absence of unequivocal hyperglycemia, this number must be confirmed by repeat testing.
Random Plasma Glucose	≥ 200 mg/dL with symptoms (Polyuria; Polydipsia; Unexplained weight loss) • Value measured without regard to last meal
Oral Glucose Tolerance Test	≥ 200 mg/dL 2 hours post 75 g glucose challenge • In absence of unequivocal hyperglycemia, this number must be confirmed by repeat testing.
Hemoglobin A1c	≥ 6 .5% • Performed in a laboratory using a method that is NGSP certified* and standardized to the DCCT assay**

 # = Fasting is defined as no caloric intake for at least 8 hours.

** National Glycohemoglobin Standardization Program; ** Diabetes Control and Complications Trial*

Practitioner may select one diagnostic tool above and in absence of unequivocal hyperglycemia should confirm results with repeat testing.

Criteria Associated with Increased Risk for Diabetes

Diagnostic Tool	Value Associated with Diagnosis of Diabetes
Impaired Fasting Glucose#	100 to 125 mg/dL
Impaired Glucose Tolerance	140 to 199 mg/dL • 2 hours post 75 g glucose challenge
Hemoglobin A1c	Range of 5.7% to 6.4%

 # = Fasting is defined as no caloric intake for at least 8 hours.

Asymptomatic patients with increased risk of diabetes who should be considered for further testing: adults of any age who are overweight or obese (BMI ≥ 25 kg/m² or BMI ≥ 23 kg/m² for Asian Americans) and who have one or more additional risk factors such as age ≥ 45. For all patients, testing should be initiated at age 45 and offered at 3-year intervals.

Updated by Jeanine P. Abrons, Elisha Andreas, and Molly Polzin

Associated Goals for Adults with Diabetes

Associated Goal	Value of Goal
Glycemic Control (A1c)	ADA*: < 7%[a] AACE**: < 6.5%[b]
Pre-Prandial Capillary Plasma Glucose	ADA: 80 to 130 mg/dL[a] AACE: < 110 mg/dL
Post-Prandial Capillary Plasma Glucose	ADA: < 180 mg/dL[a,c] AACE: < 140 mg/dL
Blood Pressure (Systolic)	ADA: < 140 mmHg[d] AACE: < 130 mmHg[e]
Blood Pressure (Diastolic)	ADA: < 90 mmHg AACE: < 80 mmHg

*American Diabetes Association (ADA) Standards of Medical Care 2018; **American Association of Clinical Endocrinologists and American College of Endocrinology Comprehensive Type 2 Diabetes Management Algorithm 2018*

a: More or less stringent glycemic goals may be appropriate for individual patients. Goals should be based on duration of diagnosis, age/life expectancy, comorbid conditions (e.g., known cardiovascular disease or advanced microvascular complications), hypoglycemia unawareness, and other considerations.

b: For patients without concurrent serious illness and at low hypoglycemic risk; level ≥ 6.5% for patients with concurrent illness and at risk for hypoglycemia. A1c targets must be individualized.

c: Post-prandial glucose may be targeted if A1c goals are not met despite reaching pre-prandial glucose goals. Measurements should be made 1-2 hours after the beginning of a meal; generally represents peak levels.

d: Lower systolic goals (e.g., < 130 mmHg) may be considered for certain individuals such as younger patients, those with albuminuria, and/or those with hypertension and one or more atherosclerotic cardiovascular disease risk factors if safe and tolerable for the patient.

e: Less stringent goals may be considered for frail patients with complicated comorbidities or those who have adverse medication effects. More intensive goal (e.g., < 120/80 mmHg) should be considered for patients if this goal can be safely reached without adverse medication-related effects.

Updated by Jeanine P. Abrons, Molly Polzin and Elisha Andreas

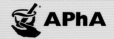

Insulin and Insulin Analogues

Type	Generic Name (Trade Name)	Onset (hours)	Peak (hours)	Duration (hours)	Administration Route
			Rapid Acting		
Analogue	Aspart (Novolog®)	0.2 to 0.3	1 to 3	3 to ≤ 5	Subcutaneous (SC) [Injection/CSII]
	Glulisine (Apidra®)	0.2 to 0.5	1.6 to 2.8		
	Lispro (Humalog®)	< 0.25	0.5 to 2.5		
			Short Acting		
Human	Regular (Humulin R®; Novolin®)	0.5	2.5 to 5	4 to 12	Daily Maintenance Use: SC [Injection/CSII]; Continuous infusion may be used in other instances
	Regular U500 (Concentrated)			Up to 24	(SC) [Injection/CSII]
			Intermediate Acting		
Human	NPH (Humulin-N®; Novolin-N®)	1 to 2	9 to 12	14 to 24	SC
			Long Acting		
Analogue; Human	Degludec (Tresiba®)	~ 1	Not applicable	Not applicable	SC
	Detemir (Levemir®)	3 to 4	3 to 9	6 to 23	
	Glargine (Lantus®)		Not applicable	10.8 to > 24	
	Glargine (Basaglar®)			≥ 24	
	Glargine (Toujeo®)	6			
			Insulin Combinations		
Combination	Degludec + Aspart (Ryzodeg® 70/30)	0.23	Not applicable	> 24	SC
	NPH + Regular (Humulin® 70/30; Novolin® 70/30)	0.5	2 to 12	18 to 24	
	Lispro protamine + Lispro (Humalog® Mix 50/50; Humalog® Mix 75/25)	0.25 to 0.5	50/50 Mix: 0.8 to 48; 75/25 Mix: 1 to 6.5	14 to 24	
	Aspart protamine + Aspart (Novolog® Mix 70/30)	0.2 to 0.3	1 to 4	18 to 24	
	Glargine + GLP-1 Agonist (Soliqua® 100/33)	Not listed	2.5 to 3	$T\frac{1}{2} = 3$ h; Clearance = 35 L/h	
	Degludec + GLP-1 Agonist (Xultophy®)		Not applicable	> 24 (see individual drugs)	

CSII = continuous subcutaneous insulin infusion
Updated by Jasmine Mangrum and Jeanine P. Abrons

Combination Oral Diabetes Medications and Insulins

Drug Class	Generic Name/ Brand Name	Dosage Range	Common Side Effects	Special Considerations/Notes ▶
COMBINATION OF CLASSES	Alogliptin + Metformin (Kazano®)*	Current dose of individual drugs to Alogliptin 25 mg/Metformin 2000 mg Daily	• Upper respiratory infection (URI)	• Dose divided twice daily with meals.
	Dapagliflozin + Metformin (Xigduo XR®)	Based upon current dose of individualized drugs: 5 mg/500 mg to 10 mg/2000 mg Daily	• Nasopharyngitis • Headache	• Dosed once daily • Fungal infection
	Glipizide + Metformin (Metaglip®)	Glipizide 2.5 mg/Metformin 250 mg or 500 mg** to 10 mg/200 mg in divided doses	• Hypoglycemia • Gastrointestinal (GI) symptoms	• Dosing based on if patient not controlled by diet/exercise alone, with a sulfonylurea &/or metformin, & fasting plasma glucose (FPG) • Start dose: no > than current daily dose of components; ↑ every 2 weeks
	Glyburide + Metformin (Glucovance®)	1.25 mg/250 mg Daily or Twice Daily** to 20 mg/2000 mg Daily With Meals		• Hypoglycemia & GI are ↑ with higher initial doses • Risk of anemia in G6PD deficiency
	Linagliptin + Metformin (Jentadueto®)	See Notes to 5 mg/2000 mg Daily		• Given in divided doses or once daily • Initial dose based on whether on metformin or not
	Pioglitazone + Metformin (Actoplus Met® Actoplus Met XR®)	**Immediate Release (IR):** Pioglitazone 15 mg/Metformin 500 to 850 mg** Daily or Twice Daily **Extended Release (ER):** Pioglitazone 15 to 30 mg/Metformin 1000 mg Daily or Twice Daily Max: Pioglitazone 45 mg/ Metformin 2000 mg Daily		• Dosing based on New York Heart Association (NYHA) heart failure (HF) class, control on metformin or pioglitazone monotherapy adequacy • Slowly ↑ based on weight gain, edema, signs/symptoms of HF • Metformin doses > 3,000 mg tolerated better if divided 3 times daily • Dose adjustment with strong CYP2C8 inhibitors • Lower extremity edema
	Repaglinide + Metformin (PrandiMet®)	See Notes to Repaglinide 10 mg/Metformin 2500 mg Daily		• Dose 2 to 3 times daily with meals • Dose based on dosing of individual drugs at start & adequacy of control • High incidence of notable side effects
	Rosiglitazone + Metformin (Avandamet®)	See Notes to Rosiglitazone 8 mg/Metformin 2000 mg		• Dose based on if patient taking individual drugs at start & adequacy of control **& should not be used with Insulin**

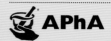

Combination Oral Diabetes Medications and Insulins *(continued)*

Drug Class	Generic Name/ Brand Name	Usual Dosage Range	Notable Side Effects	Special Considerations/Notes
COMBINATION OF CLASSES	Saxagliptin + Metformin (Kombiglyze XR®)	Use individual dose of agents to Max: 2.5 to 5 mg Saxagliptin / Metformin 1000 to 2000 mg Daily	• Headache • Diarrhea • Upper respiratory infection (URI) • Hypoglycemia • Nasopharyngitis	• Dose based on use of individual drugs, adequacy of control, or use with insulin • Dose adjustment based on use with strong CYP 3A4/5 medication
	Sitagliptin + Metformin (Janumet®, Janumet XR®))	Starting doses based on prior use of individual drugs to Sitagliptin 100 mg/Metformin 2000 mg Daily		• Dose based on use of individual drugs, adequacy of control, or use • Convert from immediate release (IR) to extended release (XR) using same total daily dose (up to max) but adjust frequency
	Rosiglitazone + Glimepiride (Avandaryl®)	Rosiglitazone 4 mg/Glimepiride 1 or 2 mg Daily to Rosiglitazone 8 mg/ Glimepiride 4 mg Daily		• Carefully titrate dose if debilitated, malnourished or in adrenal insufficiency • May take 2 weeks/2 to 3 months to see full effects
	Pioglitazone + Glimepiride (Duetact®)	Pioglitazone 30 mg/ Glimepiride 2 or 4 mg to Pioglitazone 45 mg/Glimepiride 8 mg Daily		• Dosing based on New York Heart Association (NYHA) heart failure (HF) class, control on individual drugs & adequacy of control (Causes edema/weight gain)
	Alogliptin + Pioglitazone (Oseni®)	See Notes to Alogliptin 25 mg/ Pioglitazone 45 mg Daily		• Dosing based on New York Heart Association (NYHA) heart failure (HF) class, control on individual drugs, adequacy of control on diet & exercise & insulin • Dose adjustment with strong CYP 2C8 inhibitors • Should not use if at end stage renal disease (ESRD)
	Sitagliptin + Simvastatin (Juvisync®)	Sitagliptin 100 mg/Simvastatin 40 mg**; Max: Dose of simvastatin maximum based on concurrent drug use		• Dose based on use of individual drugs, adequacy of control, or use with niacin • Maximum dose alterations: with amlodipine, amiodarone, ranolazine, diltiazem, dronedarone, verapamil, & lomitapide
	Empagliflozin + Metformin (Synjardy®)	Individualized based on patients current regimen to Empagliflozin 25 mg/ Metformin 2000 mg Daily		• Dose based on if patient taking individual drugs at start & adequacy of control or use with insulin
	Empagliflozin + Linagliptin (Glyxambi®)	Empagliflozin 10 mg/Linagliptin 5 mg to Empagliflozin 25 mg/Linagliptin 5 mg		• If present, correct volume depletion prior to initiation • Urinary tract infection (UTI)

*Note: ▶ = used for uncontrolled type 2 diabetes; * = Use alone or in combination; ** = Dose selection based upon additional criteria*

Combination Oral Diabetes Medications and Insulins *(continued)*

Drug Class	Generic Name/ Brand Names	Dosage Range	Notable Side Effects	Special Considerations/Notes
GLP-1 AGONISTS	**Exenatide** (Byetta®)	5 mcg to 10 mcg Subcutaneously Twice Daily	• Headache • Hypoglycemia • Nausea • Diarrhea • Injection site reaction	• Administer 60 minutes prior to a meal
	Exenatide Extended Release (Bydureon®)	2 mg Subcutaneously Once Weekly		• Use right away after mixing • Take with or without food
	Albiglutide (Tanzeum®)	30 mg to 50 mg Subcutaneously Once Weekly		• Take with or without food
	Dulaglutide (Trulicity®)	0.75 mg to 1.5 mg Subcutaneously Once Weekly		• Take with or without food
	Liraglutide (Victoza®)	0.6 mg Once Daily for 1 week, then ↑ to 1.2 mg Once Daily; may ↑ up to 1.8 mg Once Daily if optimal glycemic response not achevied with 1.2 mg Once Daily to Max of 1.8 mg Once Daily	**Box Warning:** Risk of developing Thyroid C-cell Tumors	• Initial starting dose is intended to reduce GI symptoms and does not provide effective glycemic control • Take with or without food • Drink non-caffeine liquids • Notable Side Effects: Tachycardia; Constipation; Vomiting

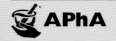

APhA

24

Oral Diabetes Medications (injectable Type 2 medications not listed) *(continued)*

Drug Class	Generic Name/ Brand Name	Usual Starting Dose	Maximum Daily Dose	Monotherapy Hypoglycemia Y/N	Notable Side Effects	Special Considerations/Notes

BIGUANIDES	**Metformin (Glucophage®)/ Metformin Oral Solution** (Riomet®)	500 mg BID to 850 mg Daily	2,550 mg daily in 2 to 3 divided doses	N	• **Black Box Warning:** Lactic Acidosis
					
					• **Other Side Effects:** GI effects
						• Contraindicated in renal dysfunction
						  • Females: Serum creatinine >1.4 mg/dL
						  • Males: Serum creatinine >1.5 mg/dL
						• Use food to lessen GI side effects

	Metformin Extended Release (Fortamet®*, Glumetza®, Glucophage XR®)	500 mg to 750 mg Daily	2,000 mg daily (*2500 mg daily)			
THIAZOLIDINEDIONES	**Pioglitazone HCl** (Actos®)**	15 mg Daily	45 mg Daily	N	• ****Black Box Warning:** Heart Failure • **Other Side Effects:** Peripheral edema Fracture May result in bladder cancer increased risk with longer use	• Contraindicated in New York Heart Association (NYHA) Class II/IV heart failure • Monitor liver function tests before and periodically with use • Safety program exists for Avandia
	Rosiglitazone Maleate (Avandia®)***	4 mg Daily or Divided	8 mg Daily, If Not On Insulin		• *****Black Box Warning:** Higher MI risk	

Updated by Jasmine Mangrum and Jeanine P. Abrons

Injectable Type 2 Diabetes Medications

Drug Class	Generic Name/Brand Name	Usual Starting Dose	Maximum Daily Dose	Notable Side Effects	Special Considerations/Notes
GLP-1 AGONISTS	Exenatide (Byetta®)	5 mcg twice daily	10 mcg twice daily	• Headache • Hypoglycemia • Nausea • Diarrhea • Injection site reaction	• Administer 60 minutes prior to a meal • Subcutaneous administration • Box warning: risk of developing thyroid C-cell tumors
	Exenatide Extended Release (Bydureon®)	2 mg once weekly	Not applicable	• Headache • Hypoglycemia • Nausea • Diarrhea • Injection site nodule	• Subcutaneous administration • Box warning: risk of developing thyroid C-cell tumors • Use right away after mixing • Take with or without food
	Albiglutide (Tanzeum®)	30 mg once weekly	50 mg once weekly	• Hypoglycemia • Diarrhea • Injection site reactions	• Subcutaneous administration • Box warning: risk of developing thyroid C-cell tumors • Take with or without food
	Dulaglutide (Trulicity®)	0.75 mg once weekly	1.5 mg once weekly	• Nausea • Diarrhea • Vomiting	• Subcutaneous administration • Box warning: risk of developing thyroid C-cell tumors • Take with or without food
	Liraglutide (Victoza®)	See notes	1.8 mg once daily	• Tachycardia • Headache • Hypoglycemia • Nausea • Constipation • Vomiting	• 0.6 mg once daily for 1 week, then increase to 1.2 mg once daily; may increase up to 1.8 mg once daily if optimal glycemic response not achieved with 1.2 mg once daily • Initial starting dose is intended to reduce GI symptoms and does not provide effective glycemic control • Subcutaneous administration • Box warning: risk of developing thyroid C-cell tumors • Take with or without food • Drink non-caffeine liquids

Prepared by Jasmine Mangrum and Jeanine P. Abrons

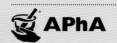
APhA

26

Initiating Therapy in Children with Intermittent Asthma Severity

Consideration	Initiating Therapy in Children with Intermittent Asthma Severity	
	Ages 0 to 4	**Ages 5 to 11**
Symptom frequency	≤ 2 days per week	≤ 2 days per week
Number of nighttime awakenings	0	2 times per month
Frequency of use of SABA to control symptoms	≤ 2 days per week	≤ 2 days per week
Extent of limitation of normal activity	No limitation	No limitation
Lung Function: • Predicted FEV_1 or personal best peak flow • FEV_1/FVC	N/A	Normal FEV_1 between exacerbations • > 80% • > 85%
Exacerbations that require oral systemic corticosteroids Considerations: severity/interval since last exacerbation	0 to 1 time per year	0 to 1 time per year
Recommended Step Therapy: Should not replace clinical decision making & individual patient needs	<u>Step 1:</u> -Re-evaluate in 2 to 6 weeks: level of asthma control -If no clear benefit in 4 to 6 weeks: stop treatment & consider another diagnosis	<u>Step 1:</u> -Re-evaluate in 2 to 6 weeks: level of asthma control -Adjust therapy accordingly

SABA = short acting beta-agonists; FEV_1 = forced expiratory volume in one second; FVC = forced vital capacity

Based on Figure 4-2a, Classifying Asthma Severity & Initiating Therapy in Children 0 to 4 Years of Age; Figure 4-2b, Classifying Asthma Severity & Initiating Treatment in Children 5 to 11 Years of Age from the National Asthma Education & Prevention Program Expert Panel Report III: Guidelines for the Diagnosis & Management of Asthma. Bethesda, MD: National Heart Lung & Blood Institute, 2007. www.nhlbi.nih.gov/guidelines/asthma/asthgdln.htm (Accessed November 2017); Global Strategy for Asthma Management & Prevention, Global Initiative for Asthma (GINA) also may be referenced. http://ginasthma.org/gina-reports/ (Accessed November 2017).

Prepared by Jeanine P. Abrons

Initiating Therapy in Children with Persistent Asthma Severity

Consideration	Initiating Therapy in Children with Persistent Asthma Severity					
	Ages 0 to 4			Ages 5 to 11		
	Mild	Moderate	Severe	Mild	Moderate	Severe
Symptom frequency	>2 days/week, but not daily	Daily	Throughout the day	>2 days/week, but not daily	Daily	Throughout the day
Number of nighttime awakenings	1 to 2 x/month	3 to 4 x/month	>1 x/week	3 to 4 x/month	>1 x/week, but not nightly	Often 7 x/week
Frequency of use of SABA to control symptoms	>2 days/week, but not daily	Daily	Several x/day	>2 days/week, but not daily	Daily	Several times/day
Extent of limitation of normal activity	Minor	Some	Extreme	Minor	Some	Extreme
Lung Function: • Predicted FEV_1, or personal best peak flow • FEV_1/FVC	N/A	N/A	N/A	• > 80% • > 80%	• 60 to 80% • 75 to 80%	• < 60% • < 75%
Exacerbations that require oral systemic corticosteroids Considerations: severity/interval since last exacerbation	≥2 in 6 months OR >4 wheezing episodes/year lasting >1 day & persistent asthma risk factors			≥ 2 x/year Relative annual risk may be related to FEV_1		
Recommended Step Therapy: Should not replace clinical decision making & individual patient needs	Step 2	Step 3 & consider short course of oral systemic corticosteroid		Step 2	Step 3: medium-dose ICS OR Step 4 and consider short course of oral systemic corticosteroids	

SABA = short acting beta-agonists; FEV_1 = forced expiratory volume in one second; FVC = forced vital capacity; ICS = inhaled corticosteroid

Based on Figure 4-2a, Classifying Asthma Severity & Initiating Therapy in Children 0 to 4 Years of Age; Figure 4-2b, Classifying Asthma Severity & Initiating Treatment in Children 5 to 11 Years of Age from the National Asthma Education & Prevention Program Expert Panel Report III: Guidelines for the Diagnosis & Management of Asthma. Bethesda, MD: National Heart Lung & Blood Institute, 2007. www.nhlbi.nih.gov/guidelines/asthma/asthgdln.htm (Accessed November 2017); Global Strategy for Asthma Management & Prevention, Global Initiative for Asthma (GINA) also may be referenced. http://ginasthma.org/gina-reports/ (Accessed November 2017).

Prepared by Jeanine P. Abrons

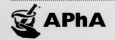

Adjusting Asthma Therapy in Children Ages 0 to 4

Consideration	Asthma Control & Therapy Adjustment (based on most impairment, risk, & recall of previous 2 to 4 weeks)		
	Well Controlled	**Not Well Controlled**	**Very Poorly Controlled**
Symptom frequency	≤ 2 days/week, but not > 1 x/day	> 2 days/week or multiple times on ≤ 2 days/week	Throughout the day
Number of nighttime awakenings	≤ 1 x/month	> 1 x/month	> 1 x/week
Frequency of use of SABA to control symptoms	≤ 2 days/week	> 2 days/week	Several x/day
Extent of limitation of normal activity	None	Some	Extreme
Lung Function: • Predicted FEV₁ or personal best peak flow • FEV₁/FVC	N/A	N/A	N/A
Exacerbations that require oral systemic corticosteroids Considerations: severity/ interval since last exacerbation	0 to 1 x/year	2 to 3 x/year	> 3 x/year
Reduction in lung growth	N/A	N/A	N/A
Treatment-related adverse effects	Side effects vary from none to troublesome; intensity does not correlate to level of control but should be considered		
Recommended Step Therapy: Should not replace clinical decision making & individual patient needs	• Maintain current step • Follow up every 1 to 6 months • Consider step down if well controlled for ≥ 3 months	• Go up 1 step	• Consider short-term course of oral systemic corticosteroid • Step up 1 to 2 steps
Considerations before step up of therapy	• Factors: adherence, inhaler technique, environmental control • If alternative therapy was used, discontinue & use preferred • Re-evaluate every 2 to 6 weeks to get control & every 1 to 6 months to maintain it • If no benefit in 4 to 6 weeks consider alternative diagnosis or therapy		

SABA = short acting beta-agonists; FEV₁ = forced expiratory volume in one second; FVC = forced vital capacity

Based on Figure 4-3a, Assessing Asthma Control & Adjusting Therapy in Children 0 to 4 Years of Age; from the National Asthma Education & Prevention Program Expert Panel Report III: Guidelines for the Diagnosis & Management of Asthma. Bethesda, MD: National Heart Lung & Blood Institute, *2007. www.nhlbi.nih.gov/guidelines/asthma/asthgdln.htm (Accessed November 2017);* Global Strategy for Asthma Management & Prevention, Global Initiative for Asthma (GINA) *also may be referenced. http://ginasthma.org/gina-reports/ (Accessed November 2017).*

Prepared by Jeanine P. Abrons

Adjusting Asthma Therapy in Children Ages 5 to 11

Consideration	Asthma Control & Therapy Adjustment (Based on most impairment, risk, & recall of previous 2 to 4 weeks)		
	Well Controlled	**Not Well Controlled**	**Very Poorly Controlled**
Symptom frequency	≤ 2 days/week, but not > 1 x/day	> 2 days/week or multiple times on ≤ 2 days/week	Throughout the day
Number of nighttime awakenings	≤ 1 x/month	≥ 2 x/month	≥ 2 x/week
Frequency of use of SABA to control symptoms	≤ 2 days/week	> 2 days/week	Several times per day
Extent of limitation of normal activity	None	Some	Extreme
Lung Function: • Predicted FEV_1 or personal best peak flow • FEV_1/FVC	 > 80% > 80%	 60 to 80% 75 to 80%	 < 60% < 75%
Exacerbations that require oral systemic corticosteroids Considerations: severity/interval since last exacerbation	0 to 1 x/year	≥ 2 x/year	≥ 2 x/year
Reduction in lung growth	Requires long-term follow up	Requires long-term follow up	Requires long-term follow up
Treatment-related adverse effects	Side effects vary from none to troublesome; intensity does not correlate to level of control but should be considered		
Recommended Step Therapy: Should not replace clinical decision making & individual patient needs	• Maintain current step • Follow up every 1 to 6 months • Consider step down if well controlled for ≥ 3 months	• Go up 1 step	• Consider short term course of oral systemic corticosteroid • Step up 1 to 2 steps
Considerations before step up of therapy	• Factors: adherence, inhaler technique, environmental control • If alternative therapy was used, discontinue & use preferred. • Re-evaluate every 2 to 6 weeks to get control & every 1 to 6 months to maintain control. • Adjust therapy accordingly.		

SABA = short acting beta-agonists; FEV_1 = forced expiratory volume in one second; FVC = forced vital capacity

Based on Figure 4-3b, Classifying Asthma Control & Adjusting Therapy in Children 5 to 11 Years of Age from the National Asthma Education & Prevention Program Expert Panel Report III: Guidelines for the Diagnosis & Management of Asthma. Bethesda, MD: National Heart Lung & Blood Institute, 2007. www.nhlbi.nih.gov/guidelines/asthma/asthgdln.htm (Accessed November 2017); Global Strategy for Asthma Management & Prevention, Global Initiative for Asthma (GINA) also may be referenced. http://ginasthma.org/gina-reports/ (Accessed November 2017).

Prepared by Jeanine P. Abrons

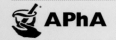

Stepwise Approach for Managing Asthma Long Term in Children Ages 0 to 4

Asthma	Step	Preferred	Alternative	Quick Relief	Notes
Intermittent	1	SABA as needed	N/A	• SABA as needed; intensity depends on symptom severity • Viral respiratory symptoms: SABA q 4 to 6h up to 24h (consider oral corticosteroid if severe) • Frequent use of SABA may mean need to step up	• This process should not replace clinical judgment. • If alternatives don't work, discontinue & use preferred. • Studies in children 0 to 4 years of age are limited.
Persistent	2	Low dose ICS	cromolyn or montelukast		
	3	Medium dose ICS	N/A		
	4	Medium dose ICS + LABA or montelukast	N/A		
	5	High dose ICS + LABA or montelukast	N/A		
	6	High dose ICS + LABA or montelukast + oral corticosteroids ICS	N/A		

SABA = short acting beta-agonists; ICS = inhaled corticosteroid; LABA = long acting beta-agonists

Stepwise Approach for Managing Asthma Long Term in Children Ages 5 to 11

Asthma	Step	Preferred	Alternative	Quick Relief	Notes
Intermittent	1	SABA as needed	N/A	• SABA as needed; intensity depends on symptom severity • SABA: up to 3 treatments at 20-minute intervals as needed • Frequent use of SABA may mean need to step up	• This process should not replace clinical judgment. • If alternatives don't work, discontinue & use preferred. • Each step: patient education, environmental control, comorbidity management • Step 2 to 4: consider allergen immunotherapy • Theophylline = less desirable
Persistent	2	Low dose ICS	cromolyn, LTRA, nedocromil, or theophylline		
	3	Low dose ICS + LABA, LTRA, or theophylline OR medium dose ICS	N/A		
	4	Medium dose ICS + LABA	Medium dose ICS + LTRA or theophylline		
	5	High dose ICS + LABA	High dose ICS + LTRA or theophylline		
	6	High dose ICS + LABA + oral corticosteroids ICS	High dose ICS + LTRA or theophylline + oral corticosteroid		

SABA = short acting beta-agonists; ICS = inhaled corticosteroid; LABA = long acting beta-agonists; LTRA = leukotriene receptor antagonist

Based on Figure 4-1a, Managing Asthma Long Term in Children 0 to 4 Years of Age: Stepwise Approach for Managing Asthma Long Term in Children, 0 to 4 Years of Age; Figure 4-1b, Managing Asthma Long Term in Children 5 to 11 Years of Age: Stepwise Approach for Managing Asthma Long Term in Children, 5 to 11 Years of Age from the National Asthma Education & Prevention Program Expert Panel Report III: Guidelines for the Diagnosis & Management of Asthma. Bethesda, MD: National Heart Lung & Blood Institute, 2007. www.nhlbi.nih.gov/guidelines/asthma/asthgdln.htm (Accessed November 2017); Global Strategy for Asthma Management & Prevention, Global Initiative for Asthma (GINA) also may be referenced. http://ginasthma.org/gina-reports/ (Accessed November 2017).

Prepared by Jeanine P. Abrons

Initiating Therapy in Youths ≥ 12 Years of Age & Adults with Intermittent Asthma Severity

Consideration	Initiating Therapy with Intermittent Asthma Severity	
	Youth ≥ 12 Years of Age & Adults	
Impairment Normal: FEV_1/FVC	Symptom frequency	≤ 2 days/week
	Number of nighttime awakenings	≤ 2 times/month
	Frequency of use of SABA to control symptoms	≤ 2 days/week
	Extent of limitation of normal activity	No limitation
	Lung Function: • Predicted FEV_1 or personal best peak flow • FEV_1/FVC	• Normal FEV_1 between exacerbations • FEV_1 > 80% predicted • FEV_1/FVC normal
Risk	**Exacerbations that require oral systemic corticosteroids** Considerations: severity & interval since last exacerbation	0 to 1 x/year
Recommendation	<u>**Recommended Step Therapy:**</u> Should not replace clinical decision making & individual patient needs	<u>Step 1:</u> Re-evaluate in 2 to 6 weeks: level of asthma control

Impairment — Normal: FEV_1/FVC

Age	Normal
8 to 19	85%
20 to 39	80%
40 to 59	75%
60 to 80	70%

SABA = short acting beta-agonists; FEV_1 = forced expiratory volume in one second; FVC = forced vital capacity

Based on Figure 4-6, Managing Asthma Long Term in Youths ≥12 Years of Age from the National Asthma Education & Prevention Program Expert Panel Report III: Guidelines for the Diagnosis & Management of Asthma. Bethesda, MD: National Heart Lung & Blood Institute, 2007. www.nhlbi.nih.gov/guidelines/asthma/asthgdln.htm (Accessed November 2017); Global Strategy for Asthma Management & Prevention, Global Initiative for Asthma (GINA) also may be referenced. http://ginasthma.org/gina-reports/ (Accessed November 2017).

Prepared by Jeanine P. Abrons

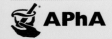

Initiating Therapy in Youths ≥ 12 Years of Age & Adults with Persistent Asthma Severity

Consideration	Initiating Therapy with Persistent Asthma Severity			
	Youth ≥ 12 Years of Age & Adults			
		Mild	Moderate	Severe
Impairment: Normal: FEV₁/FVC:	**Symptom frequency**	> 2 days/week, but not daily	Daily	Throughout the day
	Number of nighttime awakenings	3 to 4 x/month	> 1 x/week, but not nightly	Often; 7 x/week
Age / **Normal**	**Frequency of use of SABA to control symptoms**	> 2 days/week, but not daily & not > 1 x on any day	Daily	Several times/day
8 to 19 / 85%				
20 to 39 / 80%	**Extent of limitation of normal activity**	Minor limitation	Some limitation	Extreme limitation
40 to 59 / 75%	**Lung Function:** • Predicted FEV₁ or personal best peak flow • FEV₁/FVC	• FEV₁ > 80% predicted • FEV₁/FVC normal	• FEV₁ > 60% but < 80% predicted • FEV₁/FVC reduced 5%	• FEV₁ < 60% • FEV₁/FVC reduced > 5%
60 to 80 / 70%				
Risk	**Exacerbations that require oral systemic corticosteroids** Considerations: severity/interval since last exacerbation	≥ 2 x/year		
Recommendation	**Recommended Step Therapy:** Should not replace clinical decision making & individual patient needs Re-evaluate in 2 to 6 weeks: level of asthma control	Step 2	Step 3	Step 4 or 5
			Consider short course of oral systemic corticosteroids	

SABA = short acting beta-agonists; FEV₁ = forced expiratory volume in one second; FVC = forced vital capacity

Based on Figure 4-6, Managing Asthma Long Term in Youths ≥12 Years of Age from the National Asthma Education & Prevention Program Expert Panel Report III: Guidelines for the Diagnosis & Management of Asthma. Bethesda, MD: National Heart Lung & Blood Institute, 2007. www.nhlbi.nih.gov/guidelines/asthma/asthgdln.htm (Accessed November 2017); Global Strategy for Asthma Management & Prevention, Global Initiative for Asthma (GINA) also may be referenced. http://ginasthma.org/gina-reports/ (Accessed November 2017).

Prepared by Jeanine P. Abrons

Assessing Therapy in Youths ≥ 12 Years of Age & Adults Based on Asthma Control

Level of Control	Symptom Frequency	Awake at Night	Activity Limits	Symptom Control (SABA Use)	FEV₁/Peak Flow (Predicted)*	Corticosteroid Use	Treatment
Well controlled	≤ 2 days/week	≤ 2 times/month	None	≤ 2 days/week	> 80%	0 to 1 time/year	• Keep up current step & control • Follow up 1 to 6 months • Step down if control for 3 months
Not controlled	> 2 days/week	1 to 3 times/week	Some	> 2 days/week	60 to 80%	≥ 2 times/year	• 1 step up • Follow up in 2 to 6 weeks • Consider other options if side effects
Very poorly controlled	Throughout day	≥ 4 times/week	Extreme	Daily several times	< 60%	≥ 2 times/year	• May use short course of oral steroid • 1 to 2 steps up • Follow up in 2 weeks • Consider other options if side effects

SABA = short acting beta-agonists; FEV₁ = forced expiratory volume in one second; * = or personal best

FEV_1

Stepwise Approach for Managing Asthma Long Term in Youths ≥ 12 Years of Age & Adults

Asthma	Step	Preferred	Alternative or Addition	Quick Relief	Notes
Intermittent	1	SABA as needed	N/A	• SABA as needed: intensity depends on symptom severity • SABA: up to 3 treatments at 20-minute intervals as needed • Frequent use of SABA may mean need to step up	• This process should not replace clinical judgment. • If alternatives don't work, discontinue & use preferred. • Each step: patient education, environmental control, comorbidity management • Step 2 to 4: Consider allergen immunotherapy • Theophylline = less desirable
Persistent	2	Low dose ICS	**Alternative:** cromolyn, LTRA, nedocromil, or theophylline		
	3	Low dose ICS + LABA OR medium dose ICS	**Alternative:** low dose ICS + LABA, LTRA, theophylline, or zileuton		
	4	Medium dose ICS + LABA	**Alternative:** medium dose ICS + LTRA, theophylline, or zileuton		
	5	High dose ICS + LABA	**Addition:** consider omalizumab in patients with allergies		
	6	High dose ICS + LABA + oral corticosteroids	**Addition:** consider omalizumab in patients with allergies		

SABA = short acting beta-agonists; ICS = inhaled corticosteroid; LABA = long acting beta-agonist; LTRA = leukotriene receptor antagonist

Based on Figure 4-7, Assessing and Adjusting Therapy in Youths ≥12 Years of Age and Adults and on Figure 4-5, Stepwise Approach for Managing Asthma Long Term in Youths ≥12 Years of Age and Adults from the National Asthma Education & Prevention Program Expert Panel Report III: Guidelines for the Diagnosis & Management of Asthma. Bethesda, MD: National Heart Lung & Blood Institute, 2007. www.nhlbi.nih.gov/guidelines/asthma/asthgdln.htm (Accessed November 2017); Global Strategy for Asthma Management & Prevention, Global Initiative for Asthma (GINA) also may be referenced: http://ginasthma.org/gina-reports/ (Accessed November 2017).

Prepared by Jeanine P. Abrons

APhA

Assessment of Airflow Limitation/Symptoms in Chronic Obstructive Pulmonary Disease (COPD)

COPD Airflow Limitation			Symptom (Dyspnea)	
GOLD Class	Degree of Limitation	FEV$_1$*	mMRC** Grade	Description of Limitation
			0	Only gets breathless with strenuous activity
1	Mild	FEV$_1 \geq$ 80% predicted	1	Get short of breath when hurrying on level ground or walking slightly up hill
2	Moderate	50% $\leq$ FEV$_1$ < 80% predicted	2	Walks slower than others of age on level ground due to breathlessness or has to stop for breath when walking at own pace on level ground
3	Severe	30% $\leq$ FEV$_1$ < 50% predicted	3	Stops for breath when walking ~ 100 meters or after few minutes walking on level ground
4	Very Severe	FEV$_1$ < 30% predicted	4	Too breathless to leave house or when dressing or undressing

CAT^ Element	Description of Limitation
Cough	Never (0) to All the time (5)
Phlegm	None in chest (0) to Completely full of phlegm (5)
Chest Tightness	Not tight at all (0) to Very tight (5)
Hill or 1 flight of stairs	Not breathless while walking (0) to Very breathless while walking (5)
Limits Activity at Home	Not limited (0) to Very limited (5)
Confidence Leaving Home	Confident (0) to Not confident (5)
Sleeping	Sleep soundly (0) to Don't sleep soundly (5)
Energy	Have lots (0) to No energy (5) at all

*: Forced expiratory volume; Correlation between FEV$_1$, symptoms, & health status impairment is weak. Formal symptom assessment also required. Spirometric cut-points are for simplicity. To $\downarrow$ variability, perform spirometry after $\geq$ 1 dose of short-acting inhaled bronchodilator; ** mMRC: modified British Medical Research Council; ^ CAT: COPD Assessment Test; Notes: Post-bronchodilator FEV$_1$/FVC < 0.70 confirms airflow limitation; References: CAT = Jones et al. ERJ 2009;34(3):648-54; mMRC = Fletcher CM, BMJ 1960; 2017 GOLD Guidelines available at: http://goldcopd.org/gold-2017-global-strategy-diagnosis-management-prevention-copd/ (Accessed October 2017)

Use these assessments to determine ABCD Groups in COPD. From the Global Strategy for Diagnosis, Management and Prevention of COPD 2017 ©

Prepared by Jeanine P. Abrons and Anh Luong

Assessment to Determine ABCD Groups in Chronic Obstructive Pulmonary Disease (COPD)

STEP 1: Confirm Diagnosis	STEP 2: Assess Airflow Limitation/ Symptom Severity			STEP 3: Record Exacerbation History			STEP 4: Combine symptom assessment/ Exacerbation Risk	
• Use spirometry to define spirometric grade (airflow limits) • Post-bronchodilator $FEV_1/FVC < 0.70$ confirms airflow limitation	• Classify airflow limitation severity (use GOLD 1 to 4) • Assess symptoms (use mMRC Scale & CAT Assessment)			• Prior exacerbation prevalence/severity • # of prior hospitalizations/exacerbation risk:			Assessment of symptoms/risk of exacerbation	
	Class	Description		Class	Description		Gold Group	Description
With Presence of Key Indicators: • Dyspnea (progressive; worse with exercise; persistent) • Chronic cough (intermittent; unproductive; recurrent wheeze) • Chronic sputum • Recurrent lower respiratory tract infections • Family history	**Low Severity**	• mMRC ≤ 1 OR • CAT ≤ 9		**Low Risk**	0 or 1 exacerbation (not leading to hospital admission in last 12 months)		A	• Low symptom severity • Low exacerbation risk
	High Severity	• mMRC ≥ 2 OR • CAT ≥ 10		**High Risk**	≥ 2 exacerbations or any resulting in hospital admission in past 12 months		B	• High symptom severity • Low exacerbation risk
							C	• Low symptom severity • High exacerbation risk
							D	• High symptom severity • High exacerbation risk

Reference: 2017 GOLD Guidelines available at: http://goldcopd.org/gold-2017-global-strategy-diagnosis-management-prevention-copd/ (Accessed October 2017)

Prepared by Jeanine P. Abrons and Anh Luong

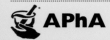

Community-Acquired Pneumonia (CAP)

Causative Bacteria	Common Signs & Symptoms	
	History of:	Physical exam findings
• S. pneumoniae	• Chalamydophila pneumoniae	• Fever
• H. influenzae	• Legionella species	• Tachypnea
• M. catarrhalis	• Mycoplasma pneumonia	• Rales OR Evidence of consolidation
	• Cough	
	• Fever & sputum production	
	• Dyspnea	
	• +/- GI symptoms	

Predisposing Factors		
• Age > 65 years	• Mechanical obstruction of bronchus	• Acidosis
• Altered consciousness	• Toxic inhalations	• Uremia
• Smoking	• Pulmonary edema	• Cystic fibrosis
• Alcohol consumption	• Bronchiectasis	• Immotile cilia syndrome
• Malnutrition	• Previous history of pneumonia	• Kartagener's syndrome
• Immunosuppression	• Chronic obstructive pulmonary disease (COPD)	• Young's syndrome
• Hypoxemia	• Age < 2 years	

How is Community Acquired Pneumonia Diagnosed?	Evaluation of Severity
• Blood cultures (x2)	• Can be made through either CURB-65 or Pneumonia Severity Index
• Chest x-ray (usually shows infiltrate)	
• Legionella: Urinary antigen assay & culture on selective media	

Note: Always consider institution specific susceptibilities
Sample References: John Hopkins Antibiotic Guide; Infectious Disease Society of America Guidelines; Albany Medical Center Hospital Formulary

Prepared by Jeanine P. Abrons

Treatment of Community-Acquired Pneumonia (CAP)

Setting/Situation	Treatment (Drug/Duration)
Outpatient (Empiric Options)	
General (Uncomplicated/No Comorbidity)	• Doxycycline for 7 to 10 days • Macrolide (Clarithromycin; Azithromycin; Erythromycin) for 7 to 10 days
With Comorbidity (COPD; Diabetes; Heart Failure) or Recent Antibiotic Therapy	• Fluoroquinolone • Beta-lactam & Macrolide: High dose Amoxicillin or Amoxicillin Clavulanate preferred; Alternatives = Ceftriaxone; Cefuroxime & Doxycycline
Hospitalized Patient (Empiric/Non-intensive Care Unit)	
Preferred (Per IDSA Guidelines)	• Fluoroquinolone (Monotherapy) for 7 to 10 days • Ceftriaxone or Cefotaxime AND Macrolide for 7 to 10 days
Aspiration Pneumonia	• Clindamycin + Fluoroquinolone • Other options: Ampicillin/Sulbactam (IV); Amoxicillin/Clavulanate (Oral) • If structural disease is present, consider pseudomonas coverage • Methicillin Resistant S. Aureus (MRSA): Add Vancomycin (Trough = 15 to 20 ug/mL or 15 mg/kg) or Linezolid
Pathogen Specific Treatment Options	
S. pneumoniae	• Amoxicillin; Ceftriaxone; Cefotaxime; Macrolide; Fluoroquinolone
MSSA	• Oxacillin; Nafcillin
Mycoplasma or Chlamydia	• Macrolide or Doxycycline for 7 days
H. influenzae	• Doxycycline; 2nd or 3rd generation Cephalosporin or Fluroquinolone x 1 to 2 weeks

*IDSA = Infectious Disease Society of America; MSSA = Methicillin Sensitive S. Aurueus

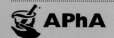

Hospital-Acquired Pneumonia Management

Common Pathogens

- ❏ **_S. Aureus_**
  - ❏ Methicillin Resistant _S. Aureus_ (MRSA)
  - ❏ Methicillin Sensitive _S. Aureus_ (MSSA)
- ❏ **Gram negative bacilli:**
  - ❏ _Klebsiella_
  - ❏ _Pseudomonas aeruginosa_
  - ❏ _Enterobacter_
  - ❏ _S. maltophilia_
  - ❏ _E. coli_
  - ❏ _Acinetobacter_ spp.
- ❏ _Legionella_ spp.
- ❏ **Gram negative bacteria:**
  - ❏ KPC (carbapenemase) producing _Klebsiella_
- ❏ **Viruses:**
  - ❏ Influenza
  - ❏ RSV
  - ❏ Parainfluenza
- ❏ **Anaerobes**

Note:
Most common are MRSA and Gram Negative Bacilli
Most difficult to treat are _P. aeruginosa_ & _Acinetobacter_

Empiric Treatment

Based on patient's risk of multi-drug resistance (MDR):
- ❏ Receipt of intravenous antibiotics during prior 90 days
- ❏ High risk of mortality

Additional risk factors for Pseudomonas:

- ❏ Hospitalization in unit where >10% of gram-negative isolates are resistant to an agent being considered for monotherapy
- ❏ Patient in septic shock
- ❏ Patient with structural lung disease (bronchiectasis; cystic fibrosis)

Additional risk factors for MRSA:

- ❏ Hospitalization in unit where >20% of _S. aureus_ isolates are methicillin resistant
- ❏ Prevalence of MRSA unknown

Note:
Refer to your institution's local susceptibilities for further guidance on empiric treatment.

Chart Based on Tables 4 and 5 of ATS/IDSA Guidelines

Empiric Therapy

NOT AT HIGH RISK of Mortality and NO FACTORS Increasing Likelihood of Multi-Drug Resistant (MDR) Pathogens (CHOOSE ONE)

Medication	Dose[a]
Piperacillin/tazobactam[b]	4.5 g IV q6h
Cefepime	2 g IV q8h
Levofloxacin	750 mg IV daily
Imipenem[b]	500 mg IV q6h
Meropenem[b]	1 g IV q8h

CHOOSE TWO for MDR and/or Pseudomonas Risk (CHOOSE ONE Beta-lactam/Carbapenem and ONE from Another Class)

Medication	Dose[a]
Piperacillin/tazobactam[b]	4.5 g IV q6h
Cefepime Ceftazidime	2 g IV q8h 2 g IV q8h
Levofloxacin Ciprofloxacin	750 mg IV daily 400 mg IV q8h
Imipenem[b] Meropenem[b]	500 mg IV q6h 1g IV q8h
Amikacin Gentamicin Tobramycin	15 to 20 mg/kg IV daily 5 to 7 mg/kg IV daily 5 to 7 mg/kg IV daily
Aztreonam	2 g IV q8h

Add for MDR and/or MRSA Risk (CHOOSE ONE)

Medication	Dose
Vancomycin	15 mg/kg IV q8 to 12h Achieve trough of 15 to 20 mg/mL (consider loading dose of 25 to 30 mg/kg IV x 1 for severe illness)
Linezolid	600 mg IV q12h

[a]Alternate dosing regimens using pharmacokinetic/pharmacodynamic (PK/PD) data may be used.
[b]Extended infusions may be appropriate.

Chart Based on Table 4 of 2016 IDSA HAP/VAP Guidelines.

Hospital-Acquired Pneumonia Management *(continued)*

HAP or VAP Suspected

Obtain lower respiratory tract (LRT) sample for culture and microscopy

Unless there is both a low clinical suspicion for pneumonia and negative microscopy of LRT sample, begin empiric antimicrobial therapy using guideline algorithm and local microbiologic data.

Day 2 & 3:
Check cultures: assess clinical response (e.g. temperature, white blood cell, chest x-ray, purulent sputum).

Clinical improvement in 48 to 72 hours

NO

Culture -	Culture +
Search for other pathogens, complications, diagnoses, or sites of infection	Adjust antibiotic therapy; search for other pathogens, complications, diagnoses, or other sites of infection

YES

Culture -	Culture +
Consider stopping antibiotics	De-escalate antibiotics (when possible). Consider treating for 7 to 8 days; then reassess.

Suggested treatment duration of 7 days

Based on Figure 1 of ATS/IDSA Guidelines

Risk Reduction:
- Effective infection control measures (education; compliance; isolation)
- Surveillance of infections to identify, quantify and prepare
- Intubation/mechanical ventilation avoidance and duration reduction when possible (guidance exists on preferred type of intubation and tubes)
- Patient positioning (semi-recumbent positioning)
- Modulation of oropharyngeal colonization by combinations of antibiotics (oral) with or without systemic therapy or selective decontamination of digestive tract (SDD)
- Consideration of risk associated with stress ulcer prophylaxis regimen or chronic proton pump inhibitor therapy
- Consideration of type of transfusion (undetermined)
- Blood glucose management

Resources:
- Institution Specific Formulary http://www.hopkinsguides.com/hopkins/ub
- Kalil AC, Metersky ML, Klompas M, Muscedere J, Sweeney DA, et al. Management of Adults with Hospital-acquired and Ventilator-associated Pneumonia: 2016 Clinical Practice Guidelines by the Infectious Diseases Society of America and the American Thoracic Society. *Clinical Infectious Diseases* 2016; 63(5):e61-111. cid.oxfordjournals.org/content/early/2016/07/06/cid.ciw353.

Prepared by Jeanine P. Abrams, Ben Lomaestro, and Bryan P. White
Additional card updates with Adrienne Rouiller

Aminoglycosides: Traditional Considerations and Dosing in Adults

General Information:

- Fight bacteria by interrupting bacterial protein synthesis.
- Bactericidal against Gram-negative aerobic organisms including Pseudomonas
- Active against Staphylococci but inactive against Streptococci
- Synergistic with some penicillins (including Ampicillin) and vancomycin against Enterococci
- Demonstrate concentration-dependent killing
- Have a significant post-antibiotic effect
- Amount in the tissue accumulates over time contributing to toxicity
- Average volume of distribution in otherwise healthy adults = 0.26 L/kg (range 0.2 to 0.3)
- Does not distribute to adipose tissue; obese patients require a correction in weight used for V_d (patients with cystic fibrosis; and ascites also may require corrections)
- Important adverse effects: Nephrotoxicity; ototoxicity; neuromuscular blockage; rash
- Elimination closely correlated with creatinine clearance

Aminoglycoside Area:	Notes/Discussion
Target Therapeutic Levels (Peaks)	• Gentamicin/Tobramycin: 4 to 8 mcg/mL (normal); Urinary tract infection: 4 to 5 mcg/mL; Endocarditis: 3 to 4 mcg/mL; Cystic fibrosis: 8 to 10 mcg/mL • Amikacin: 20 to 25 mcg/mL (Traditional Dosing); 40 to 100 mcg/mL (Single Daily Dose)
Initial or Maintenance Dose	• Doses of aminoglycosides must be individualized based on the patient characteristics such as age, weight, renal function and infection treated. • See side 2 of card for single daily dosing strategy; single daily dosing shown to have lower incidence & longer time to onset of nephrotoxicity than traditional dosing. • Gentamicin traditional dosing of adults (not single daily dosing) is 3 to 5 mg/kg IV or IM divided every 8 hours until over the age of 60 (then, 3 mg/kg divided every 12 hours) • Tobramycin traditional dosing of adults: 1 to 2 mg/kg IV over 30 minutes every 8 hours • Amikacin traditional dosing of adults: 5 mg/kg IV over 30 min every 8 hours or 7.5 mg/kg over 30 min every 12 hours • Dose adjustments must be made based on renal function. • Other certain populations also require dosage adjustments (e.g., based on post-menstrual age (Gentamicin), for cystic fibrosis, for hemodialysis (post-dialysis dosing)) • This dosing reflects adult dosing and not dosing used on neonatal or pediatric patient population.
Other Monitoring (Beyond Peak and Trough Levels)	**Monitoring Parameter** Blood Urea Nitrogen (BUN) Serum Creatinine Weight Hearing
Recommendations for Monitoring Levels	• Ensure proper timing of sampling to enable accurate interpretation of levels. Note time samples were drawn and when infusions were started and stopped. • Sampling for peak in traditional dosing completed 20 to 30 minutes following infusion; 1 hour for single daily dosing.

Prepared by Ben Lomaestro and Bryan P. White

Commonly Used Abbreviations

Term	Definition	Term	Definition
TBW	Total Body Weight	CrCl	Creatinine Clearance in mL/min
IBW	Ideal Body Weight	SCr	Serum Creatinine
NS	Normal Saline		

Aminoglycosides: Single Daily Dosing

Step	Description
1) Initial Aminoglycoside Dose given as a single daily dose (SDD):	Suggested Initial Dosing:

Drug	DOSE	
	Normal	**Critically Ill/Septic Patient**
Gentamicin	6 mg/kg	7 mg/kg
Tobramycin	6 mg/kg	7 mg/kg
Amikacin	24 mg/kg	30 to 40 mg/kg

Use TBW unless patient weight is > 40% above the IBW; then consider use of adjusted body weight or ideal body weight.

Step	Description
2) Determination of Dosing Interval	• Dosing interval is based upon estimated CrCl.

$$CrCl = \frac{(140 - age) \times IBW\ (in\ kg) \times (0.85\ in\ females)}{(72 \times SCr)}$$

• Determine the initial dosing interval:

Calculated CrCl	Initial Dosing Interval
60 mL/min or >	Every 24 hours
40 - 60 mL/min	X1 dose based on drug levels

Step	Description
3) Administration	• Administration time over 1 hour or consult institution specific guidelines. • Following infusion with a flush of 50 mL NS to ensure dose administered. • Record actual start and stop time.
4) Serum Concentration Monitoring	• Obtain PEAK concentration 1 hour after END of infusion. • Obtain a second or RANDOM concentration between 8 and 10 hours after END of infusion. • Record ACTUAL time sampled. • Record ACTUAL start and stop time of infusion and state "single dose interval." • Troughs levels should be undetectable with SDD.
5) Dosage/ Regimen Adjustment Based on Table	• Adjust dosage regimen based on serum concentrations. Dosage changes result in proportional changes in serum concentrations. PEAK (1 hour post infusion) Concentration Interpretation [Use higher level for resistant organisms]:

Drug	Recommended Action Based on PEAK Concentration	
Gentamicin and Tobramycin	Concentration	Course of Action
	7 mg/kg levels also can be evaluated based on the Hartford nomogram	
	> 25 mcg/mL	Reduce dose to achieve peak < 25 mcg/mL
	10 to 25 mcg/mL	Maintain dose
	< 10 mcg/mL	Increase dose to achieve level > 10 mcg/mL
Amikacin	Concentration	Course of Action
	> 100 mcg/mL	Reduce dose to achieve first level < 100 mcg/mL
	40 to 100 mcg/mL	Maintain dose
	< 40 mcg/mL	Increase dose to achieve level > 40 mcg/mL

• Obtaining random levels for monitoring could be considered every 8 to 12 hours. Random levels should show a decline from PEAK concentration and can be used to estimate elimination of the drug during the 24 hour dosing interval.

Nicolau DP, Freeman CD, Belliveau PP, Nightingale CH, Ross JW, Quintiliani R. Experience with a once-daily aminoglycoside program administered to 2,184 adult patients. *Antimicrob Agents Chemother.* 1995;39(3):650-5.

Use institution specific dosing guidelines if available.

Prepared by Ben Lomaestro and Bryan P. White; updated by Bryan P. White

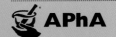

Vancomycin: Considerations and Dosing in Adults

Dosing Consideration	Notes/Discussion
Target Therapeutic Troughs	• Other Indications: 10 to 15 mcg/mL • Bacteremia, meningitis, osteomyelitis, pneumonia, endocarditis and necrotizing fasciitis: 15 to 20 mcg/mL
Initial or Maintenance Dose (For *C.difficile* Colitis Dosing—See side 2 of Card) *= Administer longer than 1 hour for doses > 1 g	• Typical dosing is based upon actual body weight. • In morbidly obese adults: Use "adjusted body weight" = *IBW + 0.4 times the difference between actual body weight and IBW (morbid obesity may be defined by kg or BMI > 40)*

Population	Dosing	
Individuals < 65 Years of Age	• **Trough Targets of 10 to 15 mcu/mL** (See Below) • **Trough Concentrations of 15 to 20 mcu/mL:** For serious infections consider loading with 20 to 30 mg/kg (May consider max 2 g/dose) IV at rate of 1 g/hour x 1. Then, 15 to 20 mg/kg IV (max 2 g/dose) at a rate 1 g/hour every 8 to 12 hours.	• **Trough Targets of 10 to 15 mcu/mL:** 15 mg/kg or 1 g intravenous (IV) every 8 to 12 hours over at least 1 hour*. Frequency Based on Renal Function. (See Below)
Individuals > 65 Years of Age	• **Trough Targets of 10 to 15 mcu/mL:** 15 mg/kg or 1 g IV over at least 1 hour.* No more often than every 12 hours initially—if CrCl < 50 mL/min give every 24 hours; If CrCl < 20 mL/min, give initial dose and base subsequent doses on drug levels. • **Trough Concentrations of 15 to 20 mcu/mL:** Consider loading with 20 to 30 mg/kg IV at a rate of 1 g/hour* then 15 to 20 mg/kg at 1 g/hour or slower at frequency adjusted for renal function (see below).	

Dose Adjustments Made Based on Renal Impairment			
> 100	Every 8 to 12 hours (If > 65 years start with every 12 hour dosing)	**10 to 19**	Every 24 to 48 hours (Monitor Levels)
80 to 99	Every 8 to 12 hours (If > 65 years start with every 12 hour dosing)	**Below 10**	750 mg to 1 g ONCE (Monitor Levels)
50 to 79	Every 12 hours	**Hemodialysis**	Based on levels and targeting trough - see reference for more information
30 to 49	Every 24 hours	**CRRT**	Single initial dose based on target and weight as above with monitoring of random levels
20 to 29	Every 24 hours		

Adverse Effects	• Rapid infusions may produce flushing or rash (Red Man's Syndrome) possibly accompanied by hypotension due to release of histamine. Slow infusions over 1 hour to reduce risk. Local reactions at site of administration; nephrotoxicity; ototoxicity; leukopenia; eosinophilia; thrombocytopenia; chills; nausea; fever muscle aches; autoimmune reactions

Notes on Use and Interpretation:
• Always refer to local institutional practices/recommendations of antimicrobial stewardship when available.
• For larger infusions administer no faster than 1 g/hour to reduce risk of red man syndrome.
• Variations in dosing may exist dependent on institution. For example, use of 2 g max loading dose.

Prepared by Ben Lomaestro and Bryan P. White

Sampling Time	Trough: 1 hour or less before next dose; Generally draw 1st trough prior to 3rd or 4th dose; trough monitoring may not accurately reflect optimal AUC exposure.

References

Crew P, Heintz SJ, Heintz BH. Vancomycin dosing and monitoring for patients with end-stage renal disease receiving intermittent hemodialysis. *Am J Health Syst Pharm.* 2015;72(21):1856-64.

Vancomycin: General Information and Dosing (PO/IV) for *C. difficile* Colitis

General Information:
Vancomycin

- Glycopeptide antimicrobial effective against gram positive organisms including *Streptococci*, *Staphylococci* (including methicillin resistant *Staphylococcus aureus* [MRSA]) and coagulase negative *Staphylococci*.

- Bacteriostatic against *Enterococci*
  Bactericidal against *Corynebacterium* and *Clostridia*.

- Use by mouth or per rectum for *C. difficile colitis*.

- Pregnancy Category: C

- Lactation: Considered Safe

- Critical drug interactions: Use caution in combining IV vancomycin with nephrotoxic or ototoxic agents such as aminoglycosides piperacillin/tazobactam, amphotericin B and cisplatin; cholestyramine and colestipol bind to vancomycin and are contraindicated when using vancomycin for *C. difficile colitis*.

C. difficile Colitis Category	Corresponding Vancomycin Dosing (From IDSA Guidelines)
Initial Episode, Mild to Moderate	• Vancomycin 125 mg by mouth every 6 hours for 10 days may be considered*; Metronidazole preferred (500 mg by mouth every 8 hours for 10-14 days.
Initial Episode, Severe	• 125 mg by mouth every 6 hours (4 times per day) for 10 to 14 days
Initial Episode, Severe/Complicated • 500 mg in 100 mL Normal Saline as a 60 min retention enema 3 to 4 times daily for 10 to 14 days	• 500 mg every 6 hours (4 times per day) by mouth or nasogastric tube plus metronidazole 500 mg every 8 hours IV. If complete ileus, consider adding rectal installation of Vancomycin.
Initial/First Recurrence	• Follow same dosing regimens as for the initial episode based on severity
Severe/Complicated or ICU	• 500 mg by mouth every 6 hours plus Metronidazole 500 mg IV every 8 hours and if patient has ileus rectal Vancomycin
Recurrent (Second and Greater)	• After acute treatment (see above) - consider taper schedule of 125 mg by mouth 2 times daily for 7 days, then 125 mg daily for 7 days, then 125 mg every 2 to 3 days for 2 to 8 weeks • Other taper regimen: 125 mg every 6 hours for 1 week; then 125 mg every 12 hours for 1 week; then 125 mg every 24 hours for 1 week; then 125 mg every 48 hours for 1 week; then 125 mg every 72 hours for 2 weeks • Pulse Therapy for Recurrent Cases: 125 to 500 mg every 2 to 3 days for 3 weeks
Clinical Definition	**Supportive Clinical Data from *C. difficile* Guidelines**
Initial episode; mild to moderate	• Leukocytosis with white blood cells (WBC) of 15,000 cells/μL or lower and SCr level <1.5 times premorbid level
Initial episode; severe	• Leukocytosis with WBCs of 15,000 cells/μL or higher and SCr ≥ 1.5 times premorbid level
Initial episode; severe complicated	• Hypotension or shock, ileus, or megacolon

Recommended Resources/References
- *C. difficile* Guidelines available at: Infectious Disease Society of America (IDSA): http://www.idsociety.org.
- Kullar R, Leonard SN, Davis SL, Delgado G, Pogue JM et al. Validation of the Effectiveness of Vancomycin Nomogram in Achieving Target Trough Concentrations of 15 to 20 mg/L Suggested by the Vancomycin Consensus Guidelines. *Pharmacotherapy*, 2011. 31(5): 441-48.
- Johnson S, Louie TJ, Gerding DN, et al. Vancomycin, metronidazole, or tolevamer for Clostridium difficile infection: results from two multinational, randomized, controlled trials. *Clin Infect Dis* 2014;59(3):345-54.
- Surawicz CM, Brandt LJ, Binion DG et al. Guidelines for diagnosis, treatment, and prevention of Clostridium difficile infections. *Am J Gastroenterol* 2013;108:478-98.

Prepared by Ben Lomaestro and Bryan P. White

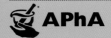

Usual Pediatric Dosages of Common Over-the-Counter (OTC) Medications

Background/Considerations:

- Over-the-counter (OTC) medications may not be labeled for use in infants or young children.
- Dosages listed represent acceptable clinical practice; dosages not listed in labeling should be given under physician guidance. Doses bolded with asterisks (*) are doses recommended for that patient group, but should be given with physician guidance.
- While age-based dosing is often available, weight-based dosing is preferred when provided. It is important to determine an accurate weight. Confirm if physician has recommended a dose to double-check dosing.
- Parents should be reminded to check expiration dates on medications at home before giving medicines to children. Doses may be recommended by the pharmacy, but the caregiver may not buy the medication because they have it at home. Instruct the parent or caregiver to check the medication strength to ensure that dosing and amounts are correct.

Administration Considerations:

- When recommending or dispensing a liquid medication, ensure the care provider has an appropriate measuring device and demonstrate how much medication to fill on the device. If a medication comes with a device, that device should be used.
- When giving a volume to the care provider to draw up, make sure to recommend a quantity that is easily measurable with the device being used, such as a dosing spoon or syringe. Marking on the syringe or providing a paper version may help to ensure recall of correct volume.
  - *Note: Per the Institute for Safe Medication Practices (ISMP) recommendations, devices should only have metric units as measurements.*
- *Parents of infants may wish to administer doses in smaller portions of the full dose at a time. This ensures that the parent will be able to quantify the amount that has been given in the event that the child spits up a portion of the medication.*
- If a child does not like the taste of the medication, it may be possible to help mask the flavor by adding the medication to other liquids (e.g., juices) or semi-solids (e.g., pudding). Check "Administration" section of package insert or a pediatric-specific drug reference to determine what is okay and what should be avoided.
  - *Note that adding medications to these substances may result in the child refusing to ingest the full amount of the medication, making it difficult to quantify the dose given.*
  - *If medication is added to other substances, use a small amount of the other substance. This ensures that all of the mixture (therefore, the full dose of the medication) can be administered as a small quantity. However, if the child wants more of the substance, additional amounts can be given without the drug.*
- If medication is given via a tube, please check with the care provider or patient to see if they can use regular oral syringes or need additional devices.

Cough/Cold/Allergy:

The Food and Drug Administration (FDA) and American Academy of Pediatrics (AAP) have issued public health advisories strongly recommending that over-the-counter (OTC) cough and cold products should not be used in infants and children less than 2 years of age. An advisory was originally issued in 2007. In 2008, voluntary removal of OTC infant products (products targeted at children less than 2 years of age) began due to safety concerns mentioned previously.

Sample Resources

· Medication Safety for Children. *Arch Pediatr Adolesc Med. 2010;* 164(2):208 in JAMA Pediatrics: Advice for Patients: (http://archpedi.jamanetwork.com/article.aspx?articleid=382713).
· https://www.fda.gov/forconsumers/consumerupdates/consumerupdatesenespanol/ucm291741.htm (Accessed 2017).
· Dundee FD, Dundee DM, Noday DM. Pediatric Counseling and Medication Management Services: Opportunities for Community Pharmacists. *J Am Pharm Assoc.* 2002; 42: 556-567.
· https://www.fda.gov/drugs/resourcesforyou/ucm133419.htm (Accessed 2017)

Prepared by Mark Botti

Pediatric Commercially Available Dosage Forms and Doses/Concentrations of Analgesics

Acetaminophen

Weight (In Pounds [lb])	Dose (In Milligrams [mg])	Dose (In milliliters [mL] of 160 mg/5 mL)
6 to 11	*40	*1.25
12 to 17	*80	*2.5
18 to 23	*120	*3.75
24 to 35	160	5
36 to 47	240	7.5
48 to 59	320	10
60 to 71	400	12.5
72 to 95	480	15

Doses can be given every 4 to 6 hours. Do not give more than 5 doses in 24 hours. Maximum daily dose is 480 mg per dose up to 5 doses, or 2400 mg total daily dose.

Liquids are available as elixir grape, cherry, berry, fruit, bubble gum, cotton candy, and strawberry. Oral disintegrating tablets are available as grape, wild grape, and bubble gum flavors. Sugar free and gluten free preparations exist. Preparations come in alcohol-free and dye-free varieties.

Ibuprofen

Weight (In Pounds [lb])	Dose (In Milligrams [mg])
Less than 12	Not recommended
12 to 17	**50***
18 to 23	**75***
24 to 35	100
36 to 47	150
48 to 59	200
60 to 71	250
72 to 95	300

Doses can be given every 6 to 8 hours. Maximum daily dose is 40 mg/kg/day up to 1200 mg/day. Maximum of 4 doses per day.

Available as an oral suspension with flavors of fruit, grape, blue-raspberry, white grape, berry, tropical punch, and bubble gum. Comes in alcohol-free, dye-free, and sugar free varieties. Chewable tabs available in grape and orange flavors.

Medication	Dosage Forms	Doses and Concentrations of Commercially Available Products
Acetaminophen	Chewable Tablets	80 mg
	Liquid	160 mg/5 mL
	Orally Disintegrating Tablets	80 mg, 160 mg
	Suppositories	80 mg, 160 mg, 325 mg, 650 mg
	Tablets/Caplets	325 mg, 500 mg, 625 mg
Ibuprofen	Capsule/Tablet	100 mg (tablet only), 200 mg
	Chewable Tablets	100 mg
	Liquids	100 mg/5 mL; 200 mg/5 mL

Doses bolded with asterisks (*) are recommended for that patient group, but should only be given with physician guidance.

Prepared by Mark Botti

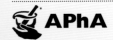

Pediatric Commercially Available Dosage Forms and Doses/Concentrations of Antihistamines

Cetirizine

Age	Dose (in milligrams [mg])	Dose (in milliliters [mL] of liquid)
< 6 months	Not recommended	Not applicable
6 to 12 months	2.5 mg once daily	2.5 mg = 2.5 mL
12 to 23 months	Initial: 2.5 mg once daily. May increase to 2.5 mg twice daily	
2 to 5 years	Initial: 2.5 mg once daily. May increase to 2.5 mg twice daily or 5 mg daily	5 mg = 5 mL
≥ 6 years	5 to 10 mg per day as one dose or divided into 2 doses	10 mg = 10 mL

Solution and syrups available as a hydrochloride are available as a liquid preparation in grape, banana-grape, and bubble gum flavor. Solutions are often dye free, gluten free, and sugar free (verify with specific product). Chewable tablets are available as tutti-fruitti, grape, and citrus.

Loratadine

Age	Dose (in milligrams [mg])	Dose (in milliliters [mL] of liquid)
< 2 years	Not recommended	Not applicable
2 to 5 years	5 mg once daily	5 mL
≥ 6 years	10 mg once daily	10 mL

Solution and syrups available as a hydrochloride are available as liquid preparations in grape, banana-grape, and fruit flavor. Chewable tablets available in grape flavor. Oral disintegrating tablets (ODT) available as bubblegum, citrus, and fruit flavors. Solutions are often alcohol free, dye free, gluten free, and sugar free (verify with specific product).

Diphenhydramine

Age (years)	Usual Dose	Max Daily Dose
< 2	Not recommended	Not applicable
2 to < 6	*6.25 to 12.5 mg	*37.5 mg/day
6-11	12.5 to 25 mg	150 mg/day
≥ 12	25 to 50 mg	300 mg/day

* Doses for 2 to < 4 years should be given under physician guidance.* Dose is 5 mg/kg/day divided into 3 to 4 doses as needed or every 4 to 8 hours. Do not take more than 6 doses/day. Comes in alcohol-free, dye-free, sorbitol-free and sugar-free options. Liquids available with cherry, fruit, berry, mango, and vanilla cherry. Strips are grape flavored. Tablets available as cherry and grape flavors.

Medication	Dosage Forms	Commercially Available Products
Cetirizine	Capsules/Dispersible Tablets	10 mg
	Chewable Tablets/Tablets	5 mg, 10 mg
	Liquid	5 mg/5 mL
Diphenhydramine	Capsules/Tablets	25 mg, 50 mg
	Chewable Tablets/Strips	12.5 mg
	Liquid	5 mg/5 mL, 12.5 mg/5 mL
Loratadine	Capsules/Tablets	10 mg
	Chewable Tablets	5 mg
	Dispersible Tablets	5 mg, 10 mg
	Liquids	5 mg/5 mL

Doses bolded with asterisks (*) are recommended for that patient group, but should only be given with physician guidance.

Prepared by Mark Botti

Pediatric Commercially Available Dosage Forms and Doses for Antiflatulents

Simethicone		
Age	**Dose (In milligrams [mg])**	**Dose (In milliliters [mL] of liquid)**
< 2 years	20	0.3
2 to 12 years	40	0.6
> 12 years	40-125; may give single dose of 500 mg; do not exceed 500 mg per day	Consider chewable tabs

Administer up to 4 times per day with meals.
Chewable tabs available in cherry crème, cool mint, peppermint, and peppermint crème. Strips available in cinnamon and peppermint. Suspension available in fruit and vanilla. Some formulations come alcohol-free, dye-free, and/or saccharin-free.

Medication	Dosage Forms	Doses/Concentrations Available
Simethicone	Capsule	125 mg, 180 mg
	Chewable Tablets	80 mg, 125 mg
	Liquids	20 mg/0.3 mL
	Strips	40 mg, 62.5 mg

Pediatric Measurements

Measuring Device	Size	Measure to Nearest:	Potential Alternative Doses
Oral Syringe*	1 mL	0.02 mL	N/A
	3 mL	0.1 mL	1.25 mL Using ¼ tsp mark
	5 mL	0.2 mL	1.25 mL, 2.5 mL, 3.75 mL Using ¼, ½, ¾ tsp marks
	10 mL	0.2 mL	2.5 mL, 7.5 mL Using ½, 1½ tsp marks
Dosing spoon	10 mL	1 mL	1.25 mL, 2.5 mL, 3.75 mL, 7.5 mL ¼, ½, ¾, 1½ tsp marks
Dosing cup	Variable	Check dosing cup	Variable

* = ISMP (Institute for Safe Medication Practices) only recommends use of oral syringes with metric doses. Other non-metric syringes not recommended.

Prepared by Mark Botti

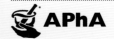

Inappropriate Medications in Older Adults

BEERS CRITERIA:

The Beers Criteria for Potentially Inappropriate Medication Use in Older Adults was originally published in 1991. Subsequent updates occurred in 1997, 2003 and 2012. The most recent updated edition was released in 2015.[1] This update removes drugs no longer available, adds new drugs and adds an expanded list of conditions considered. The new update also uses an evidence-based approach in developing the guidelines and a rating system for each criterion.

KEY POINTS:

- The criteria is not meant to substitute for professional, clinical judgment, and therapy should be individualized for each patient.
- The criteria is meant to "inform clinical decision making, research, training, and policy to improve the quality and safety of prescribing medications for older adults."[1]
- The Screening Tool of Older Persons' Potentially Inappropriate Prescriptions and Screening Tool to Alert Doctors to the Right Treatment (STOPP/START criteria) should be used in a complementary manner to the Beers Criteria.[2]

ORGANIZATION/RESOURCE:

The American Geriatrics Society (AGS) has a printable pocket card available for download on the organization's website: *http://www.geriatricscareonline.org/ProductAbstract/beers-pocket-card/PC001* (Accessed November 2017). The card organizes content from the updated Beers Criteria in extensive tables:

- Table 2: 2015 AGS Beers Criteria for Potentially Inappropriate Medication Use in Older Adults by ***Organ System/Therapeutic Category/Drug(s)***
- Table 3: 2015 AGS Beers Criteria for Potentially Inappropriate Medication Use in Older Adults Due to ***Drug-Disease or Drug-Syndrome Interactions That May Exacerbate the Disease or Syndrome***
- Table 4: Medications to Be Used with Caution
- Table 5: Clinically Important Non-anti-infective Drug-Drug Interactions
- Table 6: Non-anti-infective Medications to Avoid or Dosage Adjustments Based on Kidney Function

OTHER INFORMATION:

Most adverse drug events in older adults are attributed to a small number of medications. Four medication classes were found in a recent study to be responsible for the most adverse effects in adults: warfarin, insulin, oral antiplatelet agents, and oral hypoglycemic agents.[2,3] Close monitoring of these medication classes should be employed to reduce patient risk.

REFERENCES:

1. American Geriatrics Society 2015 Beers Criteria Update Panel. American Geriatrics Society Updated Beers Criteria for Potentially Inappropriate Medication Use in Older Adults. *J Am Geriatr Soc*, 2015. DOI: 10.1111/jgs.13702.
2. O'Mahony D, O'Sullivan D, Byrne S, et al. STOPP/START criteria for potentially inappropriate prescribing in older people: Version 2. *Age & Ageing* 2015; 44:213-18.
3. Budnitz DS, Lovegrove MC, Shehab N, Richards CL. Emergency hospitalizations for adverse drug events in older Americans. *N Engl J Med*, 2011. 365: 2002-2012.

Inappropriate Medications in Older Adults *(continued)*

Ten Medications to Avoid in Older Adults	Additional Information
1) Non-Steroidal Anti-Inflammatory Drugs (NSAIDs)	· Avoid due to risk of indigestion, ulcers, and bleeding. · Shorter acting versions are considered a safer choice. · These medications should not be taken with other medications that increase risk of bleeding.
2) Certain Diabetes Drugs	· Certain diabetes medication such as glyburide may result in hypoglycemic episodes in older adults.
3) Certain Cardiovascular Drugs	· Digoxin: avoid doses greater than 0.125 mg which can result in toxicity. · Certain blood pressure medications may increase risk of orthostatic hypotension or bradycardia. · Aspirin: evidence vs. benefit in adults 80 years of age and older. · Prasugrel: increased caution over the age of 75. · Other: warfarin, angiotensin converting enzyme inhibitors (ACEI); alpha-1 blockers; amiodarone; nifedipine; & others.
4) Muscle Relaxants	· Muscle relaxants can cause sedation, increased confusion, fall risk, constipation, dry mouth and urinary retention. · Examples include cyclobenzaprine and methocarbamol.
5) Medications for Anxiety/ Insomnia	· Medications for anxiety and insomnia can increase risk of falls and confusion.
6) Certain Anticholinergic Drugs	· Anticholinergic drugs may result in confusion, constipation, urinary retention, blurred vision, and hypotension. · Examples may include certain antidepressants, certain anti-Parkinson drugs, dicyclomine, and oxybutynin.
7) Meperidine	· This medication may cause risk of confusion and seizures.
8) Certain Antihistamine Medications	· Certain antihistamines may result in confusion, constipation, urinary retention, blurred vision, and dry mouth.
9) Antipsychotics (if not treated for psychosis)	· Haloperidol, risperidone, and quetiapine are antipsychotic medications that may result in increased risk of stroke as well as other side effects such as tremors and increased fall risk.
10) Estrogens	· Estrogens increase older adults' risk for clots and dementia.

Information adapted from Ten Medications Older Adults Should Avoid or Use with Caution. Healthinaging.org: Trusted Information. Better Care by the American Geriatrics Foundation for Health in Aging. Full content available at: http://www.healthinaging.org/files/documents/tipsheets/meds_to_avoid.pdf (Accessed November 2017).

Brief Overview of STOPP/START Criteria:
· **STOPP**: 80 clinically significant criteria for potentially inappropriate medication use (drug and disease interactions, therapeutic duplication)
· **START**: 34 common disease states in older adults where medications are indicated (evidence based)
· Organized as analgesic, cardiovascular, central nervous system, endocrine, gastrointestinal, respiratory, and urinary tract drugs.

Prepared by Jeanine P. Abrons

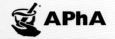

Pregnancy and Lactation Resources

Name of Resource	How to Access	Description
LactMed (Drugs and Lactation Database)	http://toxnet.nlm. nih.gov/newtoxnet/ lactmed.htm (Accessed November 2017)	· From the website: "The LactMed® database contains information on drugs and other chemicals to which breastfeeding mothers may be exposed." · Components listed: Levels anticipated; Effects in breastfed infants; Effects on Lactation and breast milk; Alternatives to consider; References · Updated monthly
Briggs' Drugs in Pregnancy and Lactation, Ninth Edition	Wolters Kluwer Health /Lippincott Williams and Wilkins Textbook; Partial (preview) version available as free download at iTunes Store	· Summarizes known/possible side effects of medications in pregnancy and possibility of passage through breast milk when nursing; A to Z searchable index · Includes: Generic name; Pharmacological class; Risk factor; Fetal risk summary; Breast feeding summary; references
Medication and a Mother's Milk	Overview: http:// www.medsmilk.com (Accessed November 2017)	· Includes recommendations by the American Academy of Pediatrics · Also includes Drug name/generic name; Uses; Drug monograph (Understood knowledge of the drug; ability to enter milk; time dependent concentration; other clinically relevant information); Pregnancy risk category; Lactation risk category; Theoretical/ relative infant dose; Adult/pediatric concerns; Drug interactions; Alternatives; Pharmacokinetic /pharmacodynamics information
Infant Risk Center	http://www.infantrisk. com (Accessed November 2017)	· Provided by Texas Tech University Health Sciences Center · Tabs on Pregnancy and Breastfeeding under "Trending Topics" · Provides general information on select topics related to pregnancy and breastfeeding

Consult multiple resources, as recommendations may differ.

Known Teratogens
Alcohol; angiotensin converting enzyme inhibitors (ACEI); Angiotensin Receptor Blockers (ARBs); Carbamazepine; Cocaine; Coumarin anticoagulants; Diethylstilbestrol (DES); Methotrexate; Phenytoin; Isotretinoin; Lithium; Misoprostol; Statins; Tetracyclines; Thalidomide; Valproate

Reference: Walters Burkey B, Holmes AP. Evaluating Medication Use in Pregnancy and Lactation: What Every Pharmacist Should Know. *J Pediatr Pharmacol Ther.* 2013; 18(3): 247-258.

Prepared by Jeanine P. Abrons

Pregnancy Risk Classifications

Risk Classification	Description
Food and Drug Administration (FDA) Drug Classification System	**Current Labeling** **New Labeling (effective June 2015)** 8.1 Pregnancy → 8.1 Pregnancy (includes Labor and Delivery) 8.2 Labor and Delivery → Merged Into 8.1 Pregnancy 8.3 Nursing Mothers → 8.2 Lactation (includes Nursing Mothers) **NEW** 8.3 Female and Males Reproductive Potential • The FDA published the "Content and Format of Labeling for Human Prescription Drug and Biological Products; Requirements for Pregnancy and Lactation Labeling" (also known as the Pregnancy and Lactation Labeling Rule) in 2014. The PLLR requires changes to content/format of prescription labeling to assist providers in determining risk versus benefit for pregnant and nursing. The law requires the label to be updated when content becomes outdated. The change went into effect June 30, 2015. Medications approved prior to June 29, 2001 are not subject to the new rule, but must have the letter category removed by June 29, 2018.
Teratogen Information System (TERIS)	• Describes risk as "unlikely," "none or minimal risk," "small to moderate," "moderate to high risk," or "risk undetermined." • Further information available at http://depts.washington.edu/terisweb/teris/ (Accessed November 2017).

Reference: http://www.fda.gov/Drugs/DevelopmentApprovalProcess/DevelopmentResources/Labeling/ucm093307.htm

Prepared by Jeanine P. Abrons

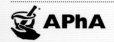

Safe and Unsafe Use of OTC Medications during Pregnancy

Common Conditions	UNSAFE OTC Treatments During Pregnancy: Trimester UNSAFE to Use	SAFE OTC Treatments During Pregnancy: Trimester SAFE to Use
Allergic Rhinitis	• Fexofenadine**(Allegra®): 1st	• **Chlorpheniramine; DOC**: all trimesters • Cetirizine (Zyrtec®): 2nd, 3rd • Loratadine (Claritin®): 2nd, 3rd
Congestion	• Phenylephrine: 1st • Pseudoephedrine: 1st	• Nasal saline sprays: all trimesters • Adhesive nasal strips: all trimesters • Use of a humidifier: all trimesters
Cough	• Guaifenesin: 1st • Codeine: all trimesters (especially 1st, 3rd)	• Dextromethorphan*: all trimesters
Pain, Fever, & Headache	• Aspirin: do not use • Ibuprofen: 3rd • Naproxen: 3rd • Aspirin/acetaminophen/caffeine (Excedrin®): do not use	• **Acetaminophen*; DOC**: all trimesters
Nausea	• Meclizine**: caution in all	• Vitamin B6^: all trimesters • Doxylamine: all trimesters • Ginger^: all trimesters
Fungal Infections & Dermatitis	• Clotrimazole: 2nd, 3rd • Miconazole: 2nd, 3rd • Tioconazole**: 2nd, 3rd	• Topical antifungals: all trimesters • Butoconazole: 2nd, 3rd • Hydrocortisone*: all trimesters
Heartburn	• Antacids: avoid doses with high amounts of calcium and aluminum	• **Calcium carbonate; DOC**: all trimesters • Omeprazole (Prilosec®): all trimesters • Antacids with Al-, Ca^{2+}, Mg^{2+}: all trimesters • Ranitidine (Zantac®) > cimetidine for chronic use: all trimesters • Famotidine (Pepcid®)**: All trimesters
Diarrhea	• Loperamide** (Imodium®): 1st • Bismuth subsalicylate (Pepto-Bismol®): do not use	• **Kaolin and pectin** (Kaopectate®); DOC**: all trimesters
Constipation	• Mineral oil: do not use • Castor oil: do not use	• **Polyethylene glycol 3350** (Miralax®); **DOC**: all trimesters
Dermatologic Disorders/Acne	• Salicylic acid (BHA) > 2%: do not use • Retinoids/retinol: do not use	• Salicylic acid (BHA) ≤ 2%: all trimesters • Benzoyl peroxide: all trimesters • Glycolic acid (AHA): all trimesters

DOC = drug of choice; PPI = proton pump inhibitors

* = recommend lowest strength for shortest time possible; ** = limited human data; ^ = herbal/vitamin supplement
This table is for general information. Always have patients discuss medications and supplements with an obstetrician. Generally, medications under "UNSAFE" have specifically been stated in literature to use with caution, to avoid in certain trimesters, to have limited human data, or to have better alternatives. Medications under "SAFE" are either DOCs, have not been cautioned for use, or do not have specific restrictions documented in literature.

References *(Accessed November 2017)*
American Academy of Family Physicians website: http://www.aafp.org/afp/2014/1015/p548.html#afp20141015p548-t3
CDC website. http://www.cdc.gov/pregnancy/meds/treatingfortwo/facts.html
American Pregnancy Association website: http://americanpregnancy.org/pregnancy-complications/cough-cold-during-pregnancy

Prepared by Brittany Hayes; updated by Jeanine P. Abrons

Immunization Schedule for Children and Adults Aged 18 Years or Younger

Vaccine	Dose/Recommended Ages for All Children	Recommended Ages for Catch-up Immunization	Other/Notes
Hepatitis B (HepB)	• 1st dose: Birth • 2nd dose: 1 month thru 2 months • 3rd dose: 6 to thru 18 months	• 4 months thru 18 years	• Minimum age: birth • Minimum interval between dose 1 & 2 = 4 weeks; • Minimum Interval between dose 2 & 3 = 8 weeks (16 weeks after 1st dose) • Minimum age for final dose = 24 weeks
Rotavirus (RV) RV₁ (2-dose series) RV₅ (3-dose series)	• 1st dose (both): 2 months • 2nd dose (both): 4 months • 3rd dose (RV5 only): 6 months	• 14 weeks 6 days = max age • 8 months = max age for final dose	• Minimum age 6 weeks for both vaccines. • If vaccine product is unknown, administer 3 doses. • Minimum interval between dose 1 & 2 = 4 weeks • Minimum interval between dose 2 & 3 = 4 weeks
Diptheria, tetanus & acellular pertussis (DTaP)	• 1st dose: 2 months • 2nd dose: 4 months • 3rd dose: 6 months • 4th dose: 15 thru 18 months • 5th dose: 4 to 6 years	• 9 months thru 4 years • 5th dose not needed if 4th dose given at ≥ age 4	• Minimum age: 6 weeks • DTaP: < 7 years • Minimum interval between dose 1 & 2; 2 & 3 = 4 weeks • Minimum interval between dose 3 & 4; 4 & 5 = 6 months
Haemophilus influenza type b (Hib)	• 1st dose: 2 months • 2nd dose: 4 months • 3rd dose*: 6 months or see booster dose • Booster dose: Age 12 thru 15 months	• Age impacted by timing of 1st dose & formulation.	• Minimum age = 6 weeks • *For ActHIB, MenHibrix, Hiberix & Pentacel • PedvaxHIB = 2 doses • For certain high risk groups: age 5 to 18 • See footnotes guidance at cdc.gov** • For minimum intervals between doses refer to cdc.gov
Pneumococcal conjugate (PCV13)	• 1st dose: 2 months • 2nd dose: 4 months • 3rd dose: 6 months • 4th dose: 12 months to 18 months	• 24-59 months (administer 1 dose to healthy children not completely vaccinated)	• Minimum age = 6 weeks • For certain high risk groups: age 5 to 18 • For minimum intervals between doses refer to cdc.gov **

** = https//www.cdc.gov/vaccines/schedules/downloads/child/0-18yrs-child-combined-schedule.pdf

Prepared by Jeanine P. Abrons and Elisha Andreas

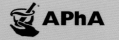

Immunization Schedule for Children and Adults Aged 18 Years or Younger *(continued)*

Vaccine	Dose/Recommended Ages for All Children	Information Related to Catch-up Immunization/Other Notes
Meningococcal Vaccines	• 1st dose of Menactra or Menveo: 11 to 12 years • 2nd dose or booster of Menactra or Menveo 16 years	• 13 to 18 years • If first dose at age 13 – 15, administer booster between age 16 thru 18 • If first dose after 16, no booster needed • Minimum ages: Hib-MenCY ≥ 6 weeks; MenACWY-D (Menactra) ≥ 9 months; MenACWY-CRM (Menveo) ≥ 2 months; MenB vaccines: 10 years • Children aged 2 months thru 18 years with high risk conditions & non-high risk groups: see CDC website • Minimum interval between dose 1 & 2 = 8 weeks
Tetanus, diphtheria & acellular pertussis (Tdap)	• 1st dose: 11 thru 12 years	• Not fully immunized with DTaP[1]: 1 dose of Tdap after age 7; if more doses needed use Td • Children 7 to 10 years dose as catch-up: additional dose at 11 thru 12 • 11 to 18 years: give 1st dose then Td booster every 10 years • Tdap minimum age = 10 years • May be administered regardless of the interval since last tetanus / diphtheria containing vaccine • Administer 1 dose in pregnancy (preferably between weeks 27 to 36) • Children age ≥ 7 years who are not fully immunized with DTaP should receive Tdap vaccine as 1 dose in catch up series. adolescent Tdap at age 11-12 may be given • Persons age 11-18 who have not gotten Tdap vaccine should receive a dose, followed by tetanus & diptheria (Td) booster dose every 10 years after. For inadvertent doses of DTaP: see CDC website
Human papillomavirus	• 2 dose series: All adolescents: Give series on schedule of 0, 6-12 months; Can start at age 9 • Administer thru age 18 • 1st dose before age 15: 2 doses on schedule of 0, 6-12 months • 1st dose at or after age 15: 3 doses on schedule of 0, 1-2, 6 months	• Vaccine dose administered at shorter intervals than minimum 2 dose schedule interval • Minimum age of 9 for 4vHPV & 9vHPV for routine/catch-up doses • Number of recommended doses based on age of administration of 1st dose • If vaccine administered on shorter interval than recommended, re-administer after minimum interval has been met • Minimum interval of 2 dose schedule: 5 months between 1st & 2nd dose; If 2nd dose administered at shorter interval, administer 3rd dose a minimum of 5 months after 1st dose • Minimum interval of 3 dose schedule: 4 weeks between 1st & 2nd dose • 12 weeks between 2nd & 3rd; 5 months between 1st & 3rd dose • See CDC site for special populations

*For Meningococcal B vaccination pneumococcal polysaccharide (PPSV23), see CDC website for use in high-risk conditions & other persons at increased risk of disease.
** = https://www.cdc.gov/vaccines/schedules/downloads/child/0-18yrs-child-combined-schedule.pdf

Prepared by Jeanine P. Abrons and Elisha Andreas

Immunizations by Age for First Year of Life

Age	Immunizations to Be Given During Normal Dosing Schedule		Needle Length / Injection Site
Birth	Hepatitis B*		Intramuscular: 5/8"; Anterolateral thigh muscle; Use 22 to 25 gauge needle
1 month	Hepatitis B (or month 2)*		Subcutaneous: 5/8" fatty tissue over anterolateral thigh muscle; Use 23 to 25 gauge needle
2 months	• Diptheria, tetanus, & acellular pertussis (DTaP < 7 years)* • Hepatitis B (or month 1)* • Haemophilus influenza type b* • Inactivated poliovirus (IPV < 18 years)	• Pneumococcal conjugate (PCV13)* • Rotavirus** • In certain high risk groups: Meningococcal*	Intramuscular: 1" in Anterolateral thigh muscle; Use 22 to 25 gauge needle
4 months	• Rotavirus** • Diptheria, tetanus, & acellular pertussis (DTaP < 7 years)* • Haemophilus influenza type b* • Pneumococcal conjugate (PCV13)*	• Inactivated poliovirus (IPV < 18 years)† • Catch up immunization potential: hepatitis B* • Certain high risk groups: Meningococcal*	
6 months	• Diptheria, tetanus, & acellular pertussis (DTaP < 7 years)* • Haemophilus influenza type b (if 3 or 4 dose series)* • Hepatitis B (potentially)* • Inactivated poliovirus (IPV < 18 years) (potentially)†	• Influenza (annually, potential)** • Pneumococcal conjugate (PCV13)* • Rotavirus (if 3 dose series)** • Certain high risk groups: Measles, mumps, rubella (MMR)***; Meningococcal*	
9 months	• Hepatitis B (potentially)* • Inactivated poliovirus (IPV < 18 years) (potentially)† • Influenza (annually, potential)**	• Catch up immunization potential: Diptheria, tetanus & acellular pertussis (DTaP < 7 years)*; Haemophilus* influenza type b; Pneumococcal conjugate (PCV13)* • Certain high risk groups: Measles, mumps, rubella (MMR)***; Meningococcal*	
12 months	• Hepatitis B (potentially)* • Haemophilus influenza type b (if 3 or 4 dose series)* • Inactivated poliovirus (IPV < 18 years) (potentially)† • Influenza (annually, potential)** • Measles, mumps, rubella (MMR) (potentially)***	• Hepatitis A (potentially)* • Pneumococcal conjugate (PCV13) (potentially)* • Varicella (potentially)*** • Catch up immunization potential: Diptheria, tetanus & acellular pertussis (DTaP < 7 years)* • Certain high risk groups: Meningococcal*	

Notes: * = Dose intramuscularly (IM) of 0.5 mL; ** = dose or route of administration & dose dependent upon product; *** = Dose subcutaneously of 0.5 mL;
† = Dose intramuscularly (IM) or subcutaneously of 0.5 mL; References: cdc.gov; immunize.org (Accessed 2018)

Prepared by Jeanine P. Abrons and Elisha Andreas

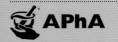

2017 Recommended Immunizations for Children from Birth Through 6 Years Old

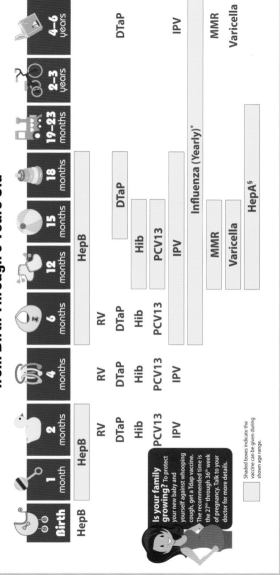

	Birth	1 month	2 months	4 months	6 months	12 months	15 months	18 months	19–23 months	2–3 years	4–6 years
HepB	HepB	HepB			HepB						
RV			RV	RV	RV						
DTaP			DTaP	DTaP	DTaP		DTaP				DTaP
Hib			Hib	Hib	Hib	Hib					
PCV13			PCV13	PCV13	PCV13	PCV13					
IPV			IPV	IPV		IPV					IPV
Influenza (Yearly)*					Influenza (Yearly)*						
MMR						MMR					MMR
Varicella						Varicella					Varicella
HepA§						HepA§					

Shaded boxes indicate the vaccine can be given during shown age range.

Is your family growing? To protect your new baby and yourself against whooping cough, get a Tdap vaccine. The recommended time is the 27th through 36th week of pregnancy. Talk to your doctor for more details.

Content source: National Center for Immunization and Respiratory Diseases.
Reference: www.cdc.gov

Travel Health Pocket Guide

	Tourists	Long-term travelers & expatriates	VFRs[a]	Humanitarian travelers	Rural travelers	Traveler's to high altitude (>8000'=2500 m)	Travelers with chronic illnesses[1,4]	Pregnant travelers[6]	Pediatric travelers	Last minute travelers	Immuno-compromised travelers[b,4]
IMMUNIZATIONS											
Age-appropriate routine vaccines[1,2]											
Hepatitis A[3]						2 doses					
Hepatitis B[4]						3 doses					
Typhoid[5]					1 injectable dose or 4 oral doses						
Yellow fever[6]						1 dose					
Rabies (pre-exposure)[7]		3 doses							3 doses		
Japanese encephalitis[8]		2 doses									
Meningococcal[9]	1 or more doses depending on indication										
Cholera[10]				1 dose							
TB testing[11]											
OTHER											
Malaria chemoprophylaxis[12]											
Traveler's diarrhea self-treatment[13]											
Acetazolamide[14]											

Legend:
- Consider for all persons in this category
- Consider if certain geographical or behavioral risk factors are present and potential benefits outweigh risks
- Generally not recommended
- No recommendation

a. Travelers who are visiting friends and/or relatives (generally defined as those returning to a home country).
b. Recommendations vary based on degree and type of immune system compromise. Severely immunocompromised patients include HIV+ with CD4 <200/mm³, asplenia, transplant recipients.

Developed by the APhA-APPM Immunizing Pharmacists Special Interest Group (SIG) Travel Committee

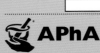

Notes:

1. **Routine vaccines:** ensure all patients are up to date on routine adult or age-appropriate pediatric vaccines, considering chronic disease diagnoses. This may include influenza (yearly), tetanus/diphtheria/pertussis, varicella, HPV, zoster, MMR, pneumococcal, polio, hepatitis A, hepatitis B, meningococcal, and Haemophilus influenza type B. Routine vaccines with travel-specific indications or considerations are discussed in further detail below. Use of the CDC catch-up immunization schedule may be necessary for pediatric patients who are un/under-vaccinated.

2. **Tetanus-containing vaccines:** consider for all patients who do not have documentation of at least one dose within the last 10 years.
   - Indicated for adults every 10 years following final pediatric dose at 11-12 years. Adults should receive a single dose of Tdap then Td every 10 years.

3. **Hepatitis A vaccination:** consider for all susceptible persons traveling to or working in countries that have high or intermediate rates of hepatitis A before traveling.
   - Persons aged ≥1 year can receive the age-appropriate dose of hepatitis A vaccine.
   - The initial dose of vaccine along with IM immune globulin at a separate injection site is recommended for the following travelers who are planning to depart to an area of risk in < 2 weeks:
     o Adults aged > 40 years, immunocompromised people, people with chronic liver disease, people with other chronic medical conditions.

4. **Hepatitis B vaccination:** consider for all unvaccinated people traveling to areas with intermediate to high prevalence of chronic hepatitis B.
   - Vaccination to prevent hepatitis B may be considered for all international travelers, regardless of destination, depending on the traveler's behavioral risk or chronic disease diagnoses.
   - Hepatitis B vaccination should begin ≥ 6 months before travel so full vaccine series can be completed before departure if possible.
     o An accelerated dosing schedule may be considered for patients at significant risk if there is not sufficient time to complete the series prior to departure.
     o For lower risk patients, 1 or 2 doses may be administered prior to departure, but optimal protection is reliable only after complete series.
   - Adult patients receiving hemodialysis or with other immunocompromising conditions: consult package insert for differences in dosing

5. **Typhoid vaccine:** consider for all patients traveling to areas of increased risk of exposure to Salmonella Typhi. Formulation choice may be based on age, patient preference and time to departure.
   - Typhim-Vi: Inactivated polysaccharide vaccine approved for patients aged ≥ 2 years. Single IM dose should be administered ≥ 2 weeks prior to possible exposure for optimal protection, but may be considered for last minute travelers. May be re-dosed every 2 years if at continued risk.
   - Vivotif: Live-attenuated oral vaccine approved for patients aged ≥ 6 years. All 4 oral capsules, taken 1 capsule every other day, should be taken for optimal protection and completed 1 week prior to possible exposure. May be re-dosed every 5 years if at continued risk.

6. **Yellow fever vaccine:** consider in those traveling to or through yellow fever endemic area or when vaccination is necessary for legal purposes. Please consult with the CDC for destination specific recommendations at http://wwwnc.cdc.gov/travel/destinations/list.
   - Yellow fever vaccine should be avoided in children < 6 months, those allergic to gelatin, latex, or egg proteins, or in those who are severely immunocompromised. HIV infection with CD4 count 200-499/mm3 is a precaution for yellow fever vaccine.
     o May offer waiver instead of vaccination when benefit does not outweigh risk.
   - Consider risk-benefit, especially in patients ≥ 60 years of age receiving first dose of yellow fever vaccine.
   - Women who are pregnant should only be vaccinated if travel to a yellow fever endemic area is unavoidable and the benefits of vaccination outweigh the risks.
   - WHO and CDC now consider a single dose to be protective for life. Country-specific regulations may still require dosing every 10 years.

Notes:

7. **Pre-exposure rabies vaccine:** consider for those who plan to or may come in contact with potentially rabid animals (e.g. rabies field workers, veterinarians, wildlife biologists, etc) and/or in those with prolonged travel or shorter stays in high risk areas (e.g. epidemic outbreaks) or with extensive outdoor stays.
   - Pre-exposure vaccination simplifies post-exposure regimen, but does not eliminate need for vaccination after exposure.
   - Rabies vaccine should not be given if time does not permit completion of series prior to departure.

8. **Japanese Encephalitis vaccine:** consider for long-term and recurrent travelers who plan to spend ≥1 month in endemic areas (Asia and parts of the Western Pacific) during the JE virus transmission season or expatriates traveling to rural or agricultural areas during a high-risk period of JE virus transmission.
   - May consider for short-term travelers (< 1 month) to endemic areas if traveling during the JE virus transmission season outside an urban area and activities will increase risk of JE virus exposure, traveling to an area with an ongoing JE outbreak or uncertain of specific destination or during peak transmission season (generally May-Dec, but may differ depending on country), activities, or duration of travel.
   - Not recommended for short-term travelers whose visits will be restricted to urban areas or times outside a well-defined JE virus transmission season.

9. **Meningococcal:** consider for patients who travel to or live in countries where meningococcal disease is hyperendemic or epidemic, including the meningitis belt of sub-Saharan Africa during the dry season (December- June). Vaccination within 3 years prior to travel required for entry into Saudi Arabia traveling to Mecca during the Hajj and Umrah pilgrimages.
   - Advisories for travelers to other at-risk countries are issued when epidemics are recognized.
   - Administer a single dose of MenACWY vaccine revaccinate with MenACWY vaccine every 5 years if the increased risk for infection remains.
   - MenB vaccine is not recommended because meningococcal disease in these countries is generally not caused by serogroup B.
   - Infants and children who received Hib-MenCY-TT are not protected against serogroups A and W and should receive a quadrivalent vaccine before traveling to areas with high endemic rates of meningococcal disease.
   - Children who received their last dose at < 7 years of age should receive an additional dose of MenACWY 3 years after their last dose.
   - Dosing schedule and number of doses dependent on age and product administered: consult package insert.

10. Cholera: consider only for adults patients from the United States to areas of active cholera transmission. Is an oral live attenuated vaccine.
    - Active cholera transmission is defined as area within a country with endemic or epidemic cholera caused by V. cholerae O1 and has had activity within the last year. Does not include areas of rare imported or sporadic cases.
    - Approved for adults 18-64 years of age. Single dose, must be administered 10 days prior to potential exposure.
    - No data exists on safety and efficacy in pregnant or breastfeeding women and immunocompromised patients.
    - Not recommended for travelers not visiting areas of active cholera transmission. Pregnant women and clinician must consider risks associated with travel to active cholera area.
    - Should not be given to patients that have taken antibiotics (oral or parenteral) in preceding 14 days.
    - If chloroquine is indicated, chloroquine must be started > 10 days after cholera vaccination.
    - Buffer of cholera vaccine may interfere with enteric coated Ty21a (Vivotif) formulation, taking first Ty21a dose > 8 hours after cholera vaccine might decrease potential interference.
    - May shed virus in stool for > 7 days, potentially may transmit to close contacts.

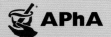

Notes:

- Requires special mixing (with supplied buffer) and consumed by patient within 15 minutes after reconstitution. Follow medical waste disposal procedures.
- Patients must avoid eating or drinking 60 minutes before and after ingestion of cholera vaccine.

11. TB testing: consider only for patients who are at increased risk of exposure during travel including healthcare workers, those who will have contact with prison or homeless populations and expatriates or long-term travelers to countries with high TB prevalence.
   - Two step tuberculin skin testing (TST) should be administered prior to travel (second test 1-3 weeks after the first) with repeat testing every 6-12 months during period of possible exposure and 8-12 weeks after return.
   - Alternative tests include interferon-gamma release assays (IGRA) which are more specific in patients who have received BCG vaccines. IGRA testing may also be used if time before departure is too short of two step TST.
   - TST may also be considered for VFR patients so as to document status prior to travel, which can aid in interpretation of future positive tests.

12. Malaria chemoprophylaxis: consider in combination with mosquito avoidance for all travelers to areas where malaria transmission occurs. Assess exact itinerary to determine patient's risk for exposure and other patient-specific factors in choosing chemoprophylaxis regimen.
   - Chloroquine and primaquine usefulness is limited to Central America, resistance exists in all other areas.
   - Avoid mefloquine in parts of South East Asia (e.g. Thailand) due to resistance.
   - Avoid mefloquine in patients with personal or family history of psychiatric diagnosis including depression and anxiety.
   - Avoid primaquine in patients who do not have documented normal G6PD levels due to risk of death due to hemolysis in deficient patients.

13. Stand-by emergency self-treatment (SBET) of traveler's diarrhea (TD): consider stand-by emergency self-treatment (SBET) for all travelers to developing countries.
   - First line antibiotics include ciprofloxacin, levofloxacin and azithromycin.
     o Fluoroquinolones should be avoided in travelers to SE Asia, as resistant strains of Camphylobacter are prevalent in countries such as Thailand.
     o Antimotilitiy agents including bismuth subsalicylate and loperimide may be recommended as adjunct symptomatic therapy.
   - Prophylactic antibiotics should not be recommended except in high-risk travelers such as those who are immunocompromised. Alternate SBET antibiotics also should be considered in addition to prophylaxis in these patients.

14. Acetazolamide altitude illness prophylaxis: consider for all travelers at moderate to high risk for altitude illness including those planning rapid ascents of more than 1,600ft (sleeping altitude) above 9,800ft with or without extra days of acclimatization every 3,300ft or those with a history of altitude illness.
   - Usual dosing is 125mg (or 250mg if >100kg) twice daily beginning 1 day prior to ascent, during ascent and for 2 days at destination altitude.

Reference: Centers for Disease Control and Prevention. CDC Heath Information for International Travel 2018. New York: Oxford University Press; 2017.

Ideal Body Weight (IBW)

Calculation	Gender/Notes	Calculation
Ideal Body Weight (in kg)	Male	50 + (2.3 x height in inches over 5 feet)
	Female	45.5 + (2.3 x height in inches over 5 feet)
	Boys ≥ 5 feet tall	39 + (2.27 x height in inches over 5 feet)
	Girls ≥ 5 feet tall	42.2 + (2.27 x height in inches over 5 feet)
	Boys & Girls < 5 feet tall	(Height^2 x 1.65)/1000

Body Mass Index (BMI)

Calculation	Gender/Notes	Calculation
Body Surface Area (BSA) (in m^2)	All	• Mosteller: $\sqrt{[\text{height (cm)} \times \text{weight (kg)}]/3600}$ • Lam: $\sqrt{[\text{height (in)} \times \text{weight (lb)}]/3131}$ • DuBois & DuBois: 0.007184 x height (cm)$^{0.725}$ x weight (kg)$^{0.425}$
Body Mass Index (BMI) (in kg/m^2)	All/ metric	• Weight (kg)/[height (m)]^2
	All/ imperial	• (Weight (lb) x 703)/height squared in (in^2)

References:
1. Mosteller RD. Simplified calculation of body-surface area [letter]. *N Engl J Med.* 1987;317(17):1098.;
2. Lam TK, Leung DT. More on simplified calculation of body surface area [letter].
   N Engl J Med. 1988;318(17):1130.;
3. DuBois D, DuBois EF. A formula to estimate the approximate surface area if height and weight be known.
   Arch Int Med. 1916;17:863–71.

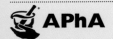

Creatinine Clearance Calculations

Name of Calculation	Formula	Appropriate Use
Cockcroft-Gault	**Women:** $= \frac{[(140 - \text{age}) \times \text{weight (in kilograms [kg])}]}{72 \times [\text{serum creatinine in mg/dL}]} \times 0.85$ **Men:** $= \frac{[(140 - \text{age}) \times \text{weight (in kilograms [kg])}]}{72 \times [\text{serum creatinine in mg/dL}]}$	❑ General use in dosing ❑ **Note:** which weight to use in the calculation is based upon the specific drug (ideal, adjusted, or actual body weight) ❑ This may require calling the company & may not be in package information. ❑ While serum creatinine may be underestimated in frail or elderly patients, it may be overestimated in muscular patients.
Schwartz	$= \frac{[\text{length in (cm)} \times k]}{\text{Serum creatinine in mg/dL}}$	❑ Used frequently in pediatric patients ❑ Presents results as mL/minute/1.73m^2
MDRD (Modified Diet in Renal Disease)	Glomerular Filtration Rate: $= 175 \times SCr^{-1.154} \times age^{-0.203}$ $\times 1.212$ (if patient is black) $\times 0.742$ (if patient is female)	Used frequently in the staging of patients Not used for acute renal failure While serum creatinine may be underestimated in frail or elderly patients, it may be overestimated in muscular patients.

Age/Classification	k value to usee
1 to 52 weeks old	0.45
1 to 13 years old	0.55
Females: 13 to 18 years old	0.55
Males: 13 to 18 years old	0.7

Recommended Resources/References

❑ Cockcroft DW, Gault MH. Prediction of creatinine clearance from serum creatinine. *Nephron*, 1976. 16(1): 31-41.

❑ Schwartz GJ, Haycock GB, Edelmann CM, Spitzer A. A simple estimate of glomerular filtration rate in children derived from body length and plasma creatinine. *Pediatrics*, 1976. 58:259-263.

❑ Levey AS, Stevens LA, Schmid CH, Zhang YL et al. A new equation to estimate glomerular filtration rate. *Ann Intern Med*, 2009. 150(9): 604-12.

Prepared by Jessica Ramich

Conversions

lb	=	kg	lb	=	kg	lb	=	kg
1		0.45	70		31.75	140		63.50
5		2.27	75		34.02	145		65.77
10		4.54	80		36.29	150		68.04
15		6.80	85		38.56	155		70.31
20		9.07	90		40.82	160		72.58
25		11.34	95		43.09	165		74.84
30		13.61	100		45.36	170		77.11
35		15.88	105		47.63	175		79.38
40		18.14	110		49.90	180		81.65
45		20.41	115		52.16	185		83.92
50		22.68	120		54.43	190		86.18
55		24.95	125		56.70	195		88.45
60		27.22	130		58.91	200		90.72
65		29.48	135		61.24			

Temperature

Fahrenheit to Centigrade or Celsius: $(°F - 32) \times 5/9 = °C$
Centigrade or Celsius to Fahrenheit: $(°C \times 9/5) + 32 = °F$

°C	=	°F	°C	=	°F	°C	=	°F
100.0		212.0	39.0		102.2	36.8		98.2
50.0		122.0	38.8		101.8	36.6		97.9
41.0		105.8	38.6		101.5	36.4		97.5
40.8		105.4	38.4		101.1	36.2		97.2
40.6		105.1	38.2		100.8	36.0		96.8
40.4		104.7	38.0		100.4	35.8		96.4
40.2		104.4	37.8		100.1	35.6		96.1
40.0		104.0	37.6		99.7	35.4		95.7
39.8		103.6	37.4		99.3	35.2		95.4
39.6		103.3	37.2		99.0	35.5		95.0
39.4		102.9	37.0		98.6	0		32.0
39.2		102.6						

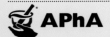
APhA

Weights and Measures

Category	Unit	Conversion
Exact Equivalents	1 ounce (oz)	28.35 grams (g)
	1 pound (lb)	453.6 g (0.4536 kilograms [kg])
	1 fluid oz (fl oz)	29.57 mL
	1 pint (pt)	473.2 mL
	1 quart (qt)	946.4 mL
Metric Conversions	1 kg	1000 g
	1 g	1000 mg
	1 mg	1000 µg
Approximate Measures: Liquids	1 fl oz	30 mL
	1 cup (8 fl oz)	240 mL
	1 pint (16 fl oz)	480 mL
	1 quart (32 fl oz)	960 mL
	1 gallon (128 fl oz)	3800 mL
Approximate Measures: Weights	1 oz	30 g
	1 lb (16 oz)	480 g
	15 grains	1 g
	1 grain	60 mg

Apothecary Equivalents

Category	Unit	Conversion
Weight	1 scruple	20 grains
	60 grains	1 dram
	8 drams	1 ounce
	1 ounce	480 grains
	16 ounces	1 pound (lb)
	1 g	15.43 grains (gr)
	1 gr	64.8 mg
	1 mg	1/65 gr
	0.8 mg	1/80 gr
	0.6 mg	1/100 gr
	0.5 mg	1/120 gr
	0.4 mg	1/150 gr
	0.3 mg	1/200 gr
	0.2 mg	1/300 gr
	0.12 mg	1/500 gr
	0.1 mg	1/600 gr
Volume	60 minims	1 fluidram
	8 fluidrams	1 fluid ounce
	1 fluid once	480 minims
	16 fluid ounces	1 pint (pt)
	1 mL	16.23 minims
	1 minim	0.06 mL

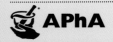

Opioid Conversions

Equianalgesic Dosing

Opioid Agonist	Oral Dose (PO)	Parenteral Dose (IV, SC, IM)	Duration of action (h)
Morphine (Immediate Release)	30 mg	10 mg	3 to 4
HYDROmorphone	7.5 mg	1.5 mg	2 to 3
OXYcodone	20 mg	---	3 to 5
HYDROcodone	30 mg	---	3 to 5
OXYmorphone	10 mg	1 mg	3 to 6
Codeine	200 mg	100 mg	4
Fentanyl	---	0.1 mg	2

Guidance for Changing Opioid Therapy

Step	Description
1	Determine the total 24-hour dose of the currently prescribed analgesic.
2	Convert the currently prescribed opioid to an equivalent morphine dose of the same route (oral vs. parenteral).
3	If the route is to remain the same, use the conversion table to convert the morphine dose to the equivalent new opioid dose. If the route is to change, first convert the morphine dose to the desired route before converting from morphine to the new opioid. · Consider decreasing dose by 50% in elderly & in patients with renal failure.
4	If pain is controlled, start at 50% to 75% of the equianalgesic dose. If pain is uncontrolled, then start at 100% of the dose.
5	Determine the strength per dose by dividing the dose calculated in Step 4 by the dosing interval. · Choose a dosing interval consistent with the medication duration of action.
6	Provide an appropriate "rescue" dose for breakthrough pain. · Ten percent of the total opioid dose given every one to two hours as needed. · Elderly: Rescue dose = 5% of the total opioid dose administered every 4 hours as needed.
7	Titrate baseline and as needed dose to provide effective pain relief.
8	Use cathartic and stool-softening medications as constipation prophylaxis.

Monitoring for Respiratory Depression
· Unintended increased sedation from opioids is a sign that the patient may be at risk for respiratory depression.

Signs of Respiratory Depression
· Respiratory rate < 10 breaths per minute
· Paradoxic rhythm with little chest expansion
· Evidence of advancing sedation
· Poor respiratory effort or quality
· Snoring or noisy respirations
· Desaturation

Prepared by Jessica Ramich

Systemic Corticosteroid Conversions

Glucocorticoid	Approximate Equivalency	Potency Relative to Hydrocortisone		Half-life T½ (Duration of Action in Hours)	Dosage Forms
		Anti-inflammatory	Mineral Corticoid		
Short Acting					
Cortisone	25 mg	0.8 mg	0.8 mg	8 to 12	PO, IM
Hydrocortisone	20 mg	1 mg	1 mg		IV, IM, PO
Intermediate Acting					
Methylprednisolone	4 mg	5 mg	0.5 mg	12 to 36	IV, IM, PO
Prednisolone	5 mg	4 mg	0.8 mg		IV, PO
Prednisone	5 mg	4 mg	0.8 mg		PO **ONLY**
Triamcinolone	4 mg	5 mg	0 mg		IM, PO
Long Acting					
Betamethasone	0.6 to 0.75 mg	20 to 30 mg	0	36 to 54	IM, PO
Dexamethasone	0.75 mg	20 to 30 mg	0	36 to 72	IV, IM, PO

PO = oral; IM = intramuscular; IV = intravenous

Suggested References

- Lexi-Drugs: Corticosteroids Systemic Equivalencies, Drug Monographs
- Facts & Comparisons: Equivalencies, Potencies, & T½, Monographs
- Micromedex: Drug Monographs
- Asare K. Diagnosis & treatment of adrenal insufficiency in the critically ill patient. *Pharmacotherapy*. 2007 Nov;27(11): 1512–28.
- Liu D, Ahmet A, Ward L, et al. A practical guide to the monitoring & management of the complications of systemic corticosteroid therapy. *Allergy, Asthma, and Clinical Immunology*. 2013. 1, 30.

Prepared by Jenna Blunt and Jeanine P. Abrons

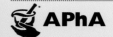

Target Serum Concentrations for Selected Drugs

Reported ranges vary according to source. Ranges reported here are for reference purposes only. Decisions regarding treatment or management of patients should be based on reference intervals reported by the specific laboratory that performs the test. Target ranges represent those for an adult population.

Drug	Target Range
Carbamazepine	4–12 µg/mL
Chloramphenicol	10–20 µg/mL (peak)　　　　　5–10 µg/mL (trough) *Note: Levels represent targets for other infections; different targets exist for meningitis*
Cyclosporine	100–400 µg/mL (blood)
Digoxin	Heart Failure–Therapeutic: 0.5–0.8 ng/mL Toxic: levels > 2ng/mL *Note: Levels should be drawn at least 6 to 8 hours after last dose, regardless of route of administration. Specific criteria exist on when to obtain concentration if loading dose is or is not given.*
Ethosuximide	40–100 µg/mL[a]
Lidocaine	Therapeutic: 1.5–5 µg/mL Toxic: > 6 µg/mL
Lithium	Therapeutic: 0.6–1.2 mEq/L Toxic: > 1.5 mEq/L *Note: Different targets exist for acute mania; prevention of episodes in patients with bipolar disorder & elderly patients.*
Phenobarbital	Infants/Children–Therapeutic: 10–40 mcg/mL Adults—Therapeutic: 10–40 µg/mL Toxic: > 40 µg/mL
Phenytoin	10–20 µg/mL[a]
Primidone	5–12 µg/mL[a]
Procainamide/ N-acetylprocainamide	Therapeutic: Procainamide: 4–10 mcg/mL; NAPA: 15–25 mcg/mL Combined: 10–30 mcg/mL
Quinidine	2–5 µg/mL[a]
Theophylline	10–20 µg/mL[a]
Valproic acid	50–100 µg/mL

[a]=Trough levels just prior to next dose

Normal Laboratory Values[a]

Chemistries

Sodium 135–146 mEq/L	Chloride 95–108 mEq/L	Blood urea nitrogen (BUN) 7–30 mg/dL	Glucose (fasting) ≤ 100 mg/dL
Potassium 3.5–5.3 mEq/L	Bicarbonate 22–29 mEq/L	Creatinine 0.5–1.5 mg/dL	

Hematology

White blood cells 3.8–10.8 × 10³/µL

Hemoglobin
13.8–17.2 g/dL (men)
12.0–15.6 g/dL (women)

Hematocrit
41%–50% (men)
35%–46% (women)

Platelets
130–400 × 10³/µL

Test	Component	Normal Range
White Blood Cell (WBC) Differential	Bands	3–5%
	Basophils	0–1%
	Eosinophils	1–3%
	Lymphocytes	23–33%
	Monocytes	3–7%
	Neutrophils	57–67%
	Segmented neutrophils (segs)	54–62%
Red Blood Cell Count	Red Blood Cell Count (Men)	4.4–5.8 x 10⁶/µL
	Red Blood Cell Count (Women)	3.9–5.2 x 10⁶/µL
MCV	Mean Corpuscular Volume (MCV)	78–102 fL
MCH	Mean Corpuscular Hemoglobin (MCH)	27–33 pg/cell
MCHC	Mean Corpuscular Hemoglobin Concentration (MCHC)	33–36%
Reticulocytes	Reticulocytes	0.5–2.3%
Arterial Blood Gasses	Base excess	±2 mEq/L
	Bicarbonate (HCO_3)	22–26 mEq/L
	Oxygen saturation	94–100%
	Partial Pressure of Carbon Dioxide ($PaCO_2$)	35–45 mmHg
	Partial Pressure of Oxygen (PaO_2)	75–100 mmHg
	pH	7.35–7.45

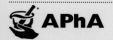

Normal Laboratory Values[a] *(continued)*

Test	Component	Normal Range
Comprehensive Metabolic Panel *See chemistries figure for additional components*	Albumin	3.5–5 g/dL
	Alkaline phosphatase (ALP)	20–125 U/L
	Bilirubin (Total)	≤ 1.3 mg/dL
	Bilirubin (Direct)	≤ 0.4 mg/dL
	Calcium (Total)	8.5–10.3 mg/dL
	Calcium (Ionized)	4.65–5.28 mg/dL
	Carbon dioxide	20–32 mEq/L
	Total Serum Protein	6.0–8.5 g/dL
Renal Function Panel*	Phosphorus	2.5–4.5 mg/dL
Uric Acid	Uric Acid (Men)	4.0–8.5 mg/dL
Enzymes	Alanine Aminotransferase (ALT)	≤ 48 U/L
	Amylase	30–170 U/L
	Aspartate aminotransferase (AST)	≤ 42 U/L
	Creatine kinase (CK) (Men)	≤ 235 U/L
	Creatine kinase (Women)	≤ 190 U/L
	Gamma glutamyltransferase (GGT) (men)	≤ 65 U/L
	GGT (women)	≤ 45 U/L
	Lactic acid dehydrogenase (LD or LDH)	≤ 270 U/L
	Lipase	7–60 u/L

[a]*Values given are for adults. Note that normal laboratory values vary widely between hospitals and laboratories; be sure to check the normal values at your site or institution.*
* See also Glucose; BUN; BUN/Creatinine Ratio; Calcium; Sodium; Potassium; Chloride; CO_2; Albumin

Fluid Composition and Calculations

Patient Monitoring Calculations

Monitoring Component	Values/Description
Serum Osmolality	$mOsm/L = (2 \times [Na^+]) + ([glucose\ in\ mg/dL]/18) + (BUN/2.8)$
Anion Gap (AGE)	$Na^+ - (Cl^- + HCO_3^-)$
Water Deficit	$0.6 \times body\ weight\ (kg) \times [1 - (140/Na^+)]$
Free Water Deficit (FWD)	Normal Total Body Weight (TBW) − Current TBW
	Normal TBW (Males) = — Lean body weight (kg) x 0.6 L/kg
	Normal TBW (Females) = — Lean body weight (kg) x 0.5 L/kg
	Current TBW = — Normal TBW (140/Current [Na^+])
Corrected Sodium	$Na^+_{measured} + [((Serum\ glucose - 100)/100) \times 1.6]$
Corrected Calcium (based on Albumin Level)	$[(Normal\ Albumin - Patient's\ Albumin) \times 0.8] + Patient's\ Measured\ total\ Ca^{2+}$
Chloride Deficit	$0.4 \times weight\ (kg) \times (100 - Cl^-_{measured})$
Bicarbonate Deficit	$(0.5 \times kg) \times (24 - HCO_3^-_{measured})$

Note: BUN = Blood Urea Nitrogen

Composition of Intravenous Fluids Used for Volume Resuscitation

Fluid Type/Fluid Component	Sodium [Na⁺] in mEq/L	Chloride (Cl⁻) in mEq/L	mOsm/L	Other
Normal Saline (0.9% NS)	154	154	308	Isotonic
5% Dextrose/0.9% NS	154	154	560	Glucose: 50 g/L
Lactated Ringers (LR)	130	109	273	Potassium: K⁺ Calcium (Ca²⁺) Lactate[1]
Dextrose 5% (5% D)	0	0	253	Glucose: 50 g/L
0.45% Normal Saline (1/2 NS)	77	77	154	
Dextrose 5%/0.45% NS	77	77	406	Glucose: 50 g/L

[1] K⁺: 4mEq/L; Ca²⁺: 1.5 mEq/L; Lactate: 28 mEq/L; Modified based on information from Merck Manual – Emergency Medicine and Critical Care – Fluid Therapy

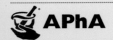

Electrolytes and Minerals

Laboratory Parameter	Normal Value
Sodium (Na⁺)	135 to 145 mEq/L
Potassium (K⁺)	3.5 to 5 mEq/L
Calcium (Ca²⁺)	8.5 to 10.5 mg/dL
Magnesium (Mg)	1.5 to 2.9 mEq/L
Phosphorus	3.7 to 4.5 mg/dL
Chloride (Cl⁻)	95 to 107 mEq/L
Bicarbonate (HCO₃⁻)	22 to 28 mEq/L
Carbon Dioxide (CO₂)	24 to 32
Blood Urea Nitrogen (BUN)	10 to 20
Serum Creatinine (SCr)	0.5 to 1 mg/dL
Glucose	65 to 99 mg/dL
White Blood Cells (WBC)	3.7 to 10.5 x 10³/µL
Hemoglobin (Hgb)	11.9 to 15.5 g/dL
Hematocrit (Hct)	35 to 47%
Platelets	150 to 400 x 10³/µL
Partial Thrombin Time (PTT)	23 to 31 seconds
Prothrombin Time (PT)	9 to 12 seconds
International Normalized Ratio (INR)	0.9 to 1.1

Note: ranges may vary based on institution-specific laboratory parameters

Psychiatry Guidelines

Topic Area/ Associated Guideline	Publication/Website	Notes
Major Depressive Disorder	American Psychiatric Association (APA). Practice guideline for the treatment of patients with major depressive disorder. 3rd ed. Arlington (VA): American Psychiatric Association (APA); 2010; http://psychiatryonline.org/pb/assets/raw/sitewide/ practiceguidelines/guidelines/mdd.pdf	Updated in 2010
Obsessive-Compulsive Disorder	American Psychiatric Association (APA). Practice guideline for the treatment of patients with obsessive-compulsive disorder. Arlington (VA): American Psychiatric Association (APA); 2007; http://psychiatryonline.org/pb/assets/raw/sitewide/ practice_guidelines/guidelines/ocd.pdf	Updated in 2007 (Guideline watch in 2013)
Generalized Anxiety Disorders	National Collaborating Centre for Mental Health, National Collaborating Centre for Primary Care. Generalised anxiety disorder and panic disorder (with or without agoraphobia) in adults. Management in primary, secondary and community care. London (UK): National Institute for Health and Clinical Excellence (NICE); 2011 Jan. 56 p. (Clinical guideline; no. 11) https://www.nice.org.uk/guidance/cg113	Updated in 2011
Panic Disorder	APA. Practice Guideline for the Treatment of Patients with Panic Disorder. 2nd ed. 2009; http://psychiatryonline.org/pb/assets/ raw/sitewide/practice_guidelines/guidelines/panicdisorder.pdf	Updated in 2009
Schizophrenia	APA Practice Guideline for the Treatment of Patients with Schizophrenia 2nd ed. http://psychiatryonline.org/pb/assets/ raw/sitewide/practice_guidelines/guidelines/schizophrenia.pdf	Updated in 2004 (Guideline watch in 2009)
Bipolar Disorder	APA Practice Guideline for the Treatment of Patients with Bipolar Disorder. http://psychiatryonline.org/pb/assets/raw/ sitewide/practice_guidelines/guidelines/bipolar.pdf	Updated in 2002 (Guideline watch 2005)

Resources for the Practicing Pharmacist

Resource	Website	Use for Pharmacy
Stahl's Essential Psychopharmacology Online	https://stahlonline.cambridge.org	Index available by drug; covers the therapeutic use and mechanisms; Guidance on how to select agents; Drug interactions; Dosing tips; Teacher images for presentation
Neuroscience Education Institute	http://neiglobal.com	Information regarding mental health pathophysiology and psychopharmacology; medication comparisons; clinical practice resources.
College of Psychiatric and Neurologic Pharmacists	http://cpnp.org	Psychiatric related job postings; Residency information; Board certification information; Continuing education resources; Suggested readings
American Psychiatric Association	http://www.psychiatry.org	Fact brochures; Several psychiatry related publications; Continuing education resources; Clinical practice resources

Prepared by Sara E. Dugan; updates with Jeanine P. Abrons

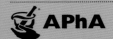

Psychiatric Medications

Medication Class	Common Adverse Drug Reactions	Clinical Pearls
Selective Serotonin Reuptake Inhibitors (SSRIs)	Somnolence; fatigue; insomnia; nausea; dry mouth; diaphoresis; sexual dysfunction; weakness (Fluoxetine); headache	Commonly utilized for the treatment of depression or anxiety disorders. Symptom improvement often takes weeks of therapy. Drug interactions due to CYP inhibition occur with some medications in this class.
Serotonin-Norepinephrine Reuptake Inhibitors (SNRIs)	Fatigue; headache; nausea; dizziness; dry mouth; insomnia; decreased appetite; hyperhidrosis (Desvenlafaxine)	Commonly utilized for the treatment of depression or anxiety disorders. Symptom improvement often takes weeks of therapy. Elevated blood pressure has been reported with some medications in this class.
Tricyclic Antidepressants (TCAs)	Weight gain; sexual dysfunction; hypotension; QT abnormalities; dry mouth; constipation; nausea; somnolence	Commonly utilized for many conditions including depression and anxiety disorders. Symptom improvement often takes weeks of therapy. Tolerability and potential toxicity are a greater concern with this class of medications.
Benzodiazepines	Sedation; dizziness; drowsiness; unsteadiness; hypotension; weakness	Commonly utilized for the treatment of agitation, anxiety, insomnia, or seizure disorders. Improvement is seen relatively quickly. These medications have the potential to cause dependence. Abrupt discontinuation may result in withdrawal seizures.
Second Generation Antipsychotics (SGA)	Sedation; dizziness; hypotension; weight gain; abnormal muscle movements; elevations in glucose or cholesterol levels	Commonly utilized for the treatment of schizophrenia and bipolar disorder, may also be used as adjunct treatment of depression. Monitoring for movement disorders is important to screen for and prevent the development of tardive dyskinesia. Regular metabolic monitoring of blood pressure, weight, glucose, and cholesterol levels is recommended.

Prepared by Sara E. Dugan

Nutrition

Harris–Benedict Equation for Basic Metabolic Rate	Ideal Body Weight Equation
Male: • 66.47 + (13.7 x kg) + (5 x cm) − (6.7 x years) = kcal/day **Female:** • 655.1 + (9.56 x kg) + (1.85 x cm) − (4.68 x years) = kcal/day **Notes:** • ↑ Metabolic requirements can be factored in by multiplying the kcal/day by an injury factor (between 1 & 2.5)	**Male:** • 50 kg + (2.3 kg x inch over 5 ft) **Female:** • 45.5 kg + (2.3 kg x inch over 5 ft)

Enteral Nutrition	
Indications for Use: "If the gut works, use it."	• Failed swallow evaluation • Esophageal mass • Intubation • Unable to meet oral (PO) intake needs • Functioning gastrointestinal (GI) tract
Sample Indications for Frequency (Duration) *Select option best for patient care*	**Continuous (24 hours)** • With initiation of enteral feeds • With labile blood sugars difficult to manage on cyclic/bolus feeds **Nocturnal or cyclic (12 to 16 hours)** • If tube feeds are used to supplement oral intake. • If TF tolerated at a higher rate: will allow more time away from feeding pump **Bolus (never an option with J-tubes)** • To simulate routine meal time schedule

Total Parenteral Nutrition (TPN)	
Indications for Use	• Non-functioning GI tract • Necessity for bowel rest • GI obstruction • GI dysfunction/malabsorption • Significant GI resection
Calculating TPN	• Weight based • Access-site dependent (central vs. peripheral) 1. Determine macronutrients 2. Determine electrolytes (based on daily labs & predicted daily requirements) 3. Determine volume/fluid needs
Ordering TPN	• Reassess electrolytes & blood sugars daily • Monitor kidney function, volume status, & current patient presentation
Weaning TPN	• ↓ rate by 50% every 20 minutes over 1 hour • Continue TPN until > 60% of PO diet is tolerated • Obtain blood glucose 1 hour after TPN is discontinued

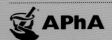

Nutrition *(continued)*

Common Daily Requirements for Parenteral Nutrition		
Component	**Standard Requirement**	**Commonly Formulated within Parenteral Nutrition Solutions**
Water	25 to 40 mL/kg	
Calcium	10 to 15 mEq	Calcium gluconate
Magnesium	8 to 20 mEq	Magnesium sulfate
Phosphorus	20 to 40 mmol	Sodium phosphate; potassium phosphate
Potassium	1 to 2 mEq/kg	Potassium chloride; potassium acetate; potassium phosphate
Sodium	1 to 2 mEq/kg	Sodium chloride; sodium acetate; sodium phosphate
Acetate	PRN to maintain acid-base balance	Sodium chloride; potassium chloride
Chloride	PRN to maintain acid-base balance	Sodium chloride; potassium chloride

Mirtallo J, Canada T, Johnson D, et al. Safe Practices for Parenteral Nutrition.
Journal of Parenteral and Enteral Nutrition, 6, S39-70. 2004.

Miscellaneous Monitoring Associated with Total Parenteral Nutrition (TPN)	
Consideration	**Information**
Albumin	3 weeks half life
Prealbumin	2 day half life
Complete metabolic panel (CMP) Complete blood counts (CBC)	Monitor daily during acute inpatient hospitalization. As patient stabilizes or goes home on TPN, labs can be done less frequently (twice weekly, weekly, or bi-weekly).
Lipid panel	Monitored frequently during acute inpatient hospitalization in patients receiving lipid emulsion therapy
Vitamins, minerals	Check if a deficiency is suspected; otherwise consider yearly
Central line infection	Patients should be educated on signs/symptoms of an infection in their central line so they can conduct daily surveillance (redness, tenderness, oozing, fever, chills, swelling, pain). If an infection is suspected, it is important that the patient seek medical attention in a timely fashion.

Sample References:

- Kreymann KG, Berger MM, Deutz NE, et al. ESPEN Guidelines on Enteral Nutrition: Intensive Care. *Clin Nutrition*, 2006. 25(2):210-23.
- Madsen H, Frankel EH. The Hitchhiker's Guide to Parenteral Nutrition Management for Adult Patients. *Practical Gastroenterology*, 2006. 46-68.
- Barnadas G. Navigating Home Care: Parenteral Nutrition – Part 2. *Practical Gastroenterology*, 2003. https://med.virginia.edu/ginutrition/wp-content/uploads/sites/199/2015/11/practicalgastro-nov03.pdf (accessed December 2017).

Calculating a TPN	
Step	**Description of Step**
1. Start by Determining Energy (Caloric) Needs	• Use the Harris–Benedict equation + Activity + stress factor = Energy (Kcal) or you may use a scale. • Sample scale: • Acute critical illness — 20 to 25 kcal/kg/day • Anabolic recovery phase — 25 to 30 kcal/kg/day • Extensive trauma or burn — 45 to 55 kcal/kg/day • Malnourished or obese — May have different caloric requirements
2. Determine Protein Needs	• High protein content may be more appropriate during the acute stages of critical illness • May start with 0.83 g/kg & add stress/other factors (e.g., 1.2 to 2.5 g/kg/day for critically ill) • To calculate grams (g) of protein supplied in a solution, multiply total volume of amino acids (in mL) by the amino acid concentration • Protein provides ~ 4 kcal/gram
3. Calculate the Fluid Needs	• Fluid needs: 25 to 35 mL/kg/day x feeding weight (kg) = Fluid needs/day (mL) = final TPN volume
4. Calculate the Fat (Lipids) Needed Based on Total Energy Needs	• Common caloric intake of available formulations: 10% fat emulsion — 1.1 kcal/mL 20% fat emulsion — 2 kcal/mL 30% fat emulsion — 3 kcal/mL • Fat: 9 kcal/gram • Fat needs: 1 to 2.5 g of fat/kg (**maximum tolerance of 2.5 g/kg feeding weight & 60% of energy [calorie content] from fat)**
5. Calculate the Carbohydrates (CHO)	• Dextrose monohydrate = 3.4 kcal/g • Determine energy content of one liter of formulation by multiplying mL x percentage of dextrose in dextrose solution • Common formulations: dextrose 50% 1 L = 500 kcal; dextrose 70% 1 L = 700 kcal • *Maximum rate of administration should not exceed 5 mg CHO/kg/min (could lead to hyperglycemia, liver dysfunction, and increase CO_2 production)* • Determine needs by subtracting fat (lipid) needs & protein calorie needs from total energy (caloric) needs. Remaining amount is needed kcal from CHO. Take kcal CHO needed/kcal per 1 L of dextrose solution = mL dextrose solution needed to make the TPN.
6. Determine Vitamin and Mineral and Other Additives	• Vitamin solutions include 12 vitamins. 10 mL dose includes: vitamin A (1 mg), vitamin D (5 mcg), vitamin E (10 mg), vitamin C (200 mg), niacinamide (40 mg), vitamin B2 (3.6 mg), vitamin B1 (6 mg), vitamin B6 (6 mg), dexpanthenol (15 mg), biotin (60 mcg), folic acid (600 mcg), & vitamin B12 (5 mcg) • Trace elements include copper, zinc, manganese, chromium, and selenium • Other additives may include insulin, H2 receptor antagonists, and iron as examples

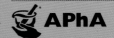

Factors to Consider When Calculating a TPN	
Factor	**Consideration**
Macronutrient Complexity	• Consider patient's ability to break down, absorb, & tolerate macronutrients
Disease Specific	• Consider whether the product is designed for a specific disease state
Obesity	• ASPEN/SCCM guidelines recommend obese patients (body mass index [BMI] >30 kg/m^2) should receive 11 to 14 kcal/kg (actual weight) or 22 to 25 kcal/kg (ideal weight); protein requirements should be dosed based upon ideal body weight (IBW)
Allergies	• Lipid emulsion products currently made from soybeans/eggs: contraindicated in patients with severe allergies to soybean/egg

ASPEN = American Society for Parenteral and Enteral Nutrition; SCCM = Society of Critical Care Medicine

Refeeding Syndrome	
Consideration	**Information**
Refeeding Syndrome General Information	• Occurs when carbohydrates are introduced to body → insulin to be released & electrolytes to be driven into cells (→ ↓ serum levels)
Risk Factors	• Body mass index (BMI) <18.5; unintentional weight loss > 10% in 3 months; little/no intake for >5 days; low electrolyte levels prior to initiation of nutrition therapy
Prevention	• Slow nutrition titration • Close electrolyte monitoring (including K$^+$, Mg^{2+}, and P$^+$) • Patients with refeeding syndrome also experience acute thiamine deficiency due to Kreb Cycle; give thiamine to at-risk patients to prevent natural depletion with administration of carbohydrates
Treatment	• Urgent repletion of electrolytes depending on the severity of lab values (including differences in dosing and formulation)

Mehanna HM, Moledina J, Travis J. Refeeding syndrome: what it is, and how to prevent and treat it. BMJ 2008; 336:1495.

Prepared by Jenna Blunt and Jeanine P. Abrons

Chronic Kidney Disease

Chronic Kidney Disease (CKD) Staging

Stage	GFR	Description	Management
Stage 1	≥ 90	Kidney damage (with normal or ↑ GFR)	Diagnosis and treatment of comorbid conditions; ↓ progression; cardiovascular risk reduction
Stage 2	60-89	Kidney damage (with mild ↓ GFR)	Estimating progression
Stage 3	30-59	Moderate ↓ GFR	Evaluating and treating complications
Stage 4	15-29	Severe ↓ GFR	Preparation for replacement therapy
Stage 5	< 15 (or dialysis)	Kidney failure	Replacement therapy by dialysis or transplantation (if uremia present)

GFR=glomerular filtration rate in mL/min/1.73m²

Management of Comorbid Conditions with CKD

Condition	Goal	Resource
Diabetes	Hgb_{A1C} ~ 7 %	National Kidney Foundation (NKF). KDOQI Clinical Practice Guideline for Diabetes & CKD: 2012 Update. *Am J Kidney Dis.* 2012 Nov;60(5):850-86.
Hypertension	< 140/90 mmHg	KDIGO Clinical Practice Guideline for the Management of Blood Pressure in CKD. *Kidney Int Suppl.* 2012 Dec;2(5):337-414.
Proteinuria	< 3 mg/mmol	KDIGO Clinical Practice Guideline for the Evaluation and Management of CKD. *Kidney Int Suppl.* 2013 Jan; 3(1):1-150.
Dyslipidemia	LDL < 100 mg/dL TG < 150 mg/dL	KDIGO Clinical Practice Guideline for Lipid Management in CKD. *Kidney Int Suppl.* 2013 Nov;3(3):259-305.
Anemia	Hgb > 11 g/dL	National Clinical Guideline Centre. Anemia Management in People with CKD. London (UK): NICE; 2011 Feb. 38.
		KDIGO Anemia Work Group. KDIGO Clinical Practice Guideline for Anemia in CKD. *Kidney Int Suppl.* 2012 Aug;2(4):279-335.
Metabolic Bone Disease	Ca^{2+}: 8.4 to 9.5 mg/dL PO^4: • 2.7 to 4.6 mg/dL (Stage 3 & 4) • 3.5 to 5.4 (Stage 5)	NICE. Hyperphosphataemia in CKD. Management of Hyperphosphataemia in Patients with Stage 4 or 5 CKD. London (UK): NICE; 2013 Mar. 22.
		KDIGO CKD-MBD Work Group. KDIGO Clinical Practice Guideline for the Diagnosis, Evaluation, Prevention, and Treatment of CKD–Mineral and Bone Disorder (MBD). *Kidney Int.* 2009 Aug; 76 (Suppl 113):S1-130.

Hgb=hemoglobin; LDL=low density lipoprotein; TG=triglycerides; KDIGO=Kidney Disease Improving Global Outcomes; NICE=National Institute for Health & Clinical Excellence

References
National Kidney Foundation Clinical Practice Guidelines for CKD: Evaluation, Classification and Stratification. New York, NY. 2002.

Johnson CA, Levey AS, Coresh J, et al. Clinical practice guidelines for chronic kidney disease in adults: Part I. Definition, disease stages, evaluation, treatment, and risk factors. *Am Fam Physician.* 2004 Sep 1;70(5):869-76.

Levey AS, Coresh J, Balk E, et al. National Kidney Foundation practice guidelines for CKD: evaluation, classification, and stratification. *Ann Intern Med.* 2003 Jul 15;139(2):137-47.

Bailie GR, Uhlig K, Levey AS. Clinical practice guidelines in nephrology: evaluation, classification, and stratification of CKD. *Pharmacotherapy.* 2005 Apr;25(4):491-502.

Prepared by Jessica Ramich

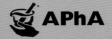

Pain Management

WHO Treatment Ladder

Step 1:
Mild to Moderate Pain
Use Non-opioid analgesics (e.g., acetaminophen, non-steroidal anti-inflammatories) ± adjuvant analgesics

Step 2:
Moderate or Persistent Pain Unrelieved by Step 1
If patient's pain is unrelieved by Step 1: Use low-dose opioid therapy ± non-opioids ± adjuvant analgesics

Step 3:
Severe or Persistent Pain Unrelieved by Step 2
If patient's pain is unrelieved by Step 2: Schedule opioids ± non-opioids ± adjuvant analgesics

Pain Assessment Tools:
- 0 to 10 Numeric Rating Scale (NRS)
- Wong-Baker FACES® Pain Rating Scale: http://wongbakerfaces.org/ (Accessed 2017)
- Visual analog scale (VAS)
- COMFORT Scale
- Face-Legs-Activity-Cry-Consolability (Pediatric)
- MOBID-2 (Dementia)

Term	Definition	Examples
Non-opioids		Acetaminophen; Ibuprofen; Naproxen; Aspirin
Opioids	Classified as weak or strong. A type of medication related to opium with analgesic properties.	Morphine, Codeine, Oxycodone, Hydromorphone, Buprenorphine, Methadone, Fentanyl
Adjuvant		Steroids, anxiolytics, antidepressants, hypnotics, anticonvulsants, sodium channel blockers, etc.

Common Adverse Effects:
Constipation, nausea/vomiting, sedation, cognitive impairment, pruritis

Other Possible Adverse Effects:
Respiratory depression, dependence, allergy

Resources:
- Schneider C, Yale SH, Larson M. Principles of Pain Management. *Clin Med Res.* 2003. 1(4): 337 to 340.
- National Institute of Health (NIH): Pain Consortium: http://painconsortium.nih.gov/index.html (Accessed 2017).
- American Academy of Pain Medicine: http://www.painmed.org/SOPResources/ClinicalTools/government-websites/ (Accessed 2017).
- JAMA Patient Page: Acute Pain Treatment. *JAMA.* 2008. 299(1): 128.
- Agency Medical Directors Group. Interagency Guideline on Opioid Dosing for Chronic Non-Cancer Pain (CNCP). 2010.
- Equianalgesic Dosing of Opioids for Pain Management. Pharmacist's Letter. August 2012.
- Gippsland Region Palliative Care Consortium Clinical Practice Group. Opioid Conversion Guidelines. February 2011.

Prepared by Jessica Ramich

Veterinary Medicine Information

Key Facts:
- Dosing usually weight based.
- More than 50% of U.S. households have a companion animal (pets are more common than children).
- Many antibiotics are available to animals as an over-the-counter (OTC) product.
- Must have a valid veterinarian-client-patient relationship.

Veterinary Consideration	Description
Differences Between Common Pets	• Dogs (canines) more commonly have hypothyroidism. • Cats (felines) more commonly have hyperthyroidism.
Counseling	**<u>Insulin Administration Technique:</u>** • Inject at a 45° angle under skin around neck of a dog or cat (e.g., where a mom cat carries her kittens). • Keep needle parallel to skin & inject under loose skin between neck & back. • Subcutaneous is preferred; intramuscular (IM) administration is an option (administer IM in thigh) but not preferred due to nerve damage risk ○ Further details: http://www.peteducation.com (accessed December 2017) **<u>SIG Abbreviations:</u>** • Vary for humans & animals (e.g., Once daily: Humans = QD; Animals = SID)
Dosing Considerations	• Pain medications/antibiotics dosed higher & more often (different from humans).

Toxicity	• Ingestion (accidental or overdose) of some OTC products may be toxic to pets.
	   ○ Acetaminophen Example: Cat (feline) toxic dose = > 10 mg/kg; Dog (Canine) = > 200 mg/kg
	      ○ Treatment: N-acetylcysteine; Cimetidine within 48 hours

Compounding	• FDA Regulations & Compliance Policy Guide 608.400 "Compounding of Drugs for Use in Animals." • For a compounding prescription to be valid for a pet, a valid relationship must exist between provider & patient (pet/owner) • Veterinary medicines may be compounded when no approved animal or human drug is available. • A beyond-use date should be assigned as indicated for the product.

Drug, Dosing, & Pharmacology Resources

- National Animal Poison Control Center: www.aspca.org/pet-care/poison-control
- Plumb's Veterinary Drug Handbook
- American Veterinary Medical Association - Compounding: https://www.avma.org/KB/Policies/Pages/Compounding.aspx

Veterinary Disease States

- Petplace.com
- Peteducation.com

Legal & Regulatory Resources

- Food & Drug Association (FDA)/Center for Veterinary Medicine (CVM): http://www.fda.gov/AnimalVeterinary

Prepared by Breanna Sunderman

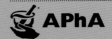

Quality, Free Online Resources

Resource	Features or Benefit	Limitations in Use
U.S. Food and Drug Administration http://www.fda.gov/	• Animal Drugs®FDA (Green Book) • Therapeutic Equivalence Evaluations (Orange Book) • Drugs®FDA • FDA Drug Shortages • National Drug Code Directory	The large amount of information may make navigation difficult.
U.S. National Library of Medicine https://www.nlm.nih.gov/	• MEDLINE/PubMed/MedlinePlus • ClinicalTrials.gov • DailyMed • Pillbox • Populations and genetics information • Environmental health & toxicology	The connection or overlap of information between libraries; cross-referencing is improving.
Drugs.com https://www.drugs.com	• ~24,000 monographs from Wolters Kluwer Health, American Society of Health-System Pharmacists, Cerner Multum, & Micromedex from Truven Health	This website may appear cluttered. Commercial advertising is accepted.
Medscape: Drugs & Diseases http://reference.medscape.com	• ~ 7,100 monographs based on FDA approvals	Information is abbreviated & may not be comprehensive.
Merck Manuals http://www.merckmanuals.com/	• Drug monographs from Wolters Kluwer Clinical Drug Information, Inc. • Consumer/Professional Version • Veterinary Edition	Publication reflects medical practice & information in the United States. It does not include international perspectives.
Centers for Disease Control and Prevention http://www.cdc.gov/	• Morbidity & Mortality Weekly Report • Free travel apps: TravWell; Can I Eat This?; 2016 Yellow Book	Lots of information but easy navigation.
Drug Enforcement Administration (DEA) https://www.dea.gov	• Drugs of Abuse	Focused on enforcement of controlled substances laws & US Regulations; not global.
World Health Organization http://www.who.int/en/	• International Pharmacopoeia • World Health Report • International Travel & Health • International Classification of Diseases-10	The website's expansive coverage makes navigation difficult.
Institute for Safe Medication Practices (ISMP) http://www.ismp.org	• ISMP Guidelines • Medication Error Reporting • Medication safety tools and resources	The organization provides independent oversight. It relies on donations & grants. Subscriptions are fee-based.
Agency for Healthcare Research and Quality (AHRQ) http://www.ahrq.gov/	• National Guideline Clearinghouse • Health Literacy Center	Lots of information but easy to navigate.

All sites accessed November 2017
Prepared by Jeanine P. Abrons

National Clinical Guidelines

Cardiovascular Section Guidelines

Guideline (Publication Date)	Recognized Source of Guideline
Antithrombotic and Thrombolytic Therapy (2016)	American College of Chest Physicians (CHEST)
ASCVD (2013)	American College of Cardiology and American Heart Association (ACC/AHA)
Heart Failure (2017) **Acute (2014); Chronic (2010)**	American College of Cardiology, American Heart Association, and Heart Failure Society of America (ACC/AHA/HFSA) National Institute for Health and Care Excellence (NICE)
Hypertension (2017)	American College of Cardiology and American Heart Association (ACC/AHA)
Lifestyle Management to Reduce Cardiovascular Risk (2013)	American College of Cardiology and American Heart Association (ACC/AHA)
Myocardial Infarction (MI) (2013/2014/2015)	American College of Cardiology and American Heart Association (ACC/AHA)
Overweight and Obesity (2013)	American College of Cardiology, American Heart Association, The Obesity Society (ACC/AHA/TOS)
Stroke (2018) **Guidelines also exist for prevention**	American Heart Association and American Heart Association (AHA/ASA)

Endocrine Section Guidelines

Guideline (Publication Date)	Recognized Source of Guideline
Diabetes (2018)	American Diabetes Association (ADA)
Endocrine (multiple years)	American Association of Clinical Endocrinologists and American College of Endocrinology (AACE/ACE)

Respiratory Section Guidelines

Guideline (Publication Date)	Recognized Source of Guideline
Asthma (GINA 2017)	Global Initiative for Asthma (GINA)
Chronic Obstructive Pulmonary Disease (2017)	Global Initiative for Chronic Obstructive Lung Disease (GOLD)

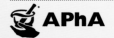

National Clinical Guidelines *(continued)*

Infectious Diseases Section Guidelines

Guideline (Publication Date)	Where to Access
Community Acquired Pneumonia (CAP) (2007) Projected update Spring 2018	Infectious Diseases Society of America
Hospital Acquired Pneumonia (HAP) (2016)	Infectious Diseases Society of America
C. Difficile **(2010)** Projected update Fall 2017	Infectious Diseases Society of America
Other (multiple years)	Infectious Diseases Society of America

Special Populations Section Guidelines

Guideline (Publication Date)	Where to Access
Beers Criteria (2015)	American Geriatrics Society
Pharmacological Management of Persistent Pain in Older Persons (2009)	American Geriatrics Society
Prevention of Falls in Older Persons (2010)	American Geriatrics Society

Miscellaneous Section Guidelines

Guideline (Publication Date)	Where to Access
General	
National Guideline Clearinghouse (multiple years)	http://www.guideline.gov
Mental Health	
Alzheimer's Disease (2011)	https://www.alz.org/health-care-professionals/clinical-guidelines-dementia-care.asp

Prepared by Jeanine P. Abrons

Clinically Significant Drug Interactions

Category/ Classification	Electronic Resource
Cytochrome P450 Drug Interactions	Indiana University Division of Clinical Pharmacology P450 Drug Interaction Table *(http://medicine.iupui.edu/clinpharm/ddis/main-table/)*
QTc Prolonging Medications	Arizona Center for Education and Research on Therapeutics *(https://www.crediblemeds.org/index.php/login/dlcheck)* Free Registration now required
Grapefruit Interactions with Medications	Center for Drug Interaction and Education Research *(http://www.druginteractioncenter.org)* FDA *(http://www.fda.gov/ForConsumers/consumerupdates/ ucm292276.htm)*
General Interactions including Herbals	University of Maryland Drug Interaction Checker *(http://umm.edu/health/medical/drug-interaction-tool)*
Oral Contraception Interactions/ Pregnancy	Reprotox *(http://www.reprotox.org/Default.aspx)* Additional resources listed in "Special Populations" section
Herbal Information	National Center for Complementary and Alternative Medicine *(http://nccam.nih.gov/health/ herbsataglance.htm)*
Dietary Supplements	National Center for Complementary and Alternative Medicine *(http://nccam.nih.gov/health/supplements/ wiseuse.htm)*

All websites accessed December 2017   *Prepared by Jeanine P. Abrons*

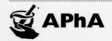

Medications with Adverse Withdrawal Effects from Abrupt Discontinuation – SEVERE to MODERATE

Medication Category	Medication Examples	Presentation with Abrupt Stop	Symptoms	Management/Risk Factors	Evidence	Potential to be Life Threatening
Anticoagulant	Rivaroxaban (Xarelto®) Apixaban (Eliquis®) Dabigatran (Pradaxa®) Edoxaban (Savaysa®) Warfarin (Coumadin®)	↑ risk of thrombotic events	Severe	• If stopped for reasons other than bleeding or therapy end, consider another anticoagulant	Excellent	YES
Anticonvulsant	Gabapentin (Neurotin®) Pregabalin (Lyrica®) Phenytoin (Dilantin®)	Seizures; Anxiety; Insomnia; Nausea; Pain; Sweating	Mild to Severe	• **Management:** · Taper over at least 2 to 4 weeks	Good	YES
Antiparkinson	Carbidopa/Levodopa (Sinemet®) Amantadine (Symmetrel®) Rasagiline (Azilect®)	Hyperpyrexia; Confusion; Muscle rigidity; Tachycardia; Tachypnea	Severe	• **Management:** · Taper over ~ 4 weeks	Good	YES
Alpha Agonist	Clonidine (Catapres®)	Rebound hypertension; Tachycardia; Agitation; Headache; Stroke (rarely): Encephalopathy (rarely)	Mild to Severe	• **Management:** · Taper over 1 to 2 weeks • **Risk factors:** use > 1 month, cardiovascular disease, beta-blocker use, daily dose > 1.2 mg	Excellent	YES
Antipsychotic	Clozapine (Clozaril®) Quetiapine (Seroque®) Olanzapine (Zyprexa®) Risperidone (Risperdal®) Haloperidol (Haldol®)	Sweating; Salivation; Flu symptoms; Paresthesia; Bronchoconstriction; Urination; gastrointestinal; Anorexia; Vertigo; Insomnia, Agitation/ anxiety; Restlessness; Movement disorders, Psychosis	Mild to Severe	• **Management:** · No > 50% ↓ every 2 weeks. · May stop more abruptly in hospital. · If switching agent, may cross-taper: ↓ dose of old agent while titrating up new agent at ~ same rate (e.g., over 2 to 3 weeks)	Excellent	NO
Beta blocker	Atenolol (Tenormin®) Bisoprolol (Zebeta®) Metoprolol (multiple)) Propranolol (Inderal®)	Hypertension; Angina; Myocardial Infarction, Ventricular Arrhythmia	Mild to Severe	• **Management:** · ↓ dosage over 1 to 2 weeks & up to 3 weeks with history of myocardial infarction	Good	YES

Updated by Angela Wojtczak, Joanna Rusch, Elisha Andreas, and Jeanine P. Abrons.

Medications with Adverse Withdrawal Effects from Abrupt Discontinuation – MODERATE

Medication Category	Medication Examples	Presentation with Abrupt Stop	Symptoms	Management/Risk Factors	Evidence	Potential to be Life Threatening
Benzodiazepine & "Z drugs"	Alprazolam (Xanax®) Clonazepam (Klonopin®) Lorazepam (Ativan®) Triazolam (Halcion) Eszopiclone (Lunesta) Zolpidem (Ambien)	Sweating; Tremor; Agitation; Nausea; Tachycardia; Insomnia Anxiety; Vomiting; Hallucinations; Seizures	Mild to Severe	• **Risk factors:** · High-dose, long-term use · Use of short acting agent • **Management:** · Taper or sub long-acting agent over 2 to 3 months	Excellent	YES
Butalbital combination products	Fiorinal Fioricet	Headache exacerbation; Delirium; Tremors; Seizures	Mild to Severe	• **Risk factors:** · Constant, long-term use of ≥ 7 doses daily • **Management:** · Taper over 4 to 6 weeks. With ≥ 12 doses daily, consider referral.	Fair	YES
Corticosteroid	Prednisone (Deltasone®) Methylprednis (Solu-Medrol®) Hydrocortisone (Cortef®)	Adrenal insufficiency - Nausea; Vomiting; Fatigue; Weakness, ↓ Appetite; ↓ Weight; Hypoglycemia; ↓ Mood; Adrenal Crisis	Mild to Severe	• **Risk factor:** · Prednisone > 7.5 mg daily for > 3 weeks • **Management:** · Based on institution; Taper over 2 months for pituitary-adrenal response recovery	Excellent	YES
Nitrate	Isosorbide mononitrate & dinitrate (Imdur®, Isordil®)	Rebound angina	Mild to Severe	• **Management:** · Consider taper over 1 to 2 weeks use sublingual nitroglycerine as needed	Fair – Good	NO
Opioid	Oxycodone (OxyContin®) Hydrocodone (Hysingla®) Codeine Morphine (MS Contin®)	Flu-like symptoms; Insomnia; Anxiety; Cramps; Fatigue; Malaise	Mild to Severe	• **Management:** · Taper over 2 to 3 weeks if severe adverse effects, overdose, or with abuse. · Taper by ≤ 10% of original dose per week.	Good	NO

Updated by Angela Wojtczak, Joanna Rusch, Elisha Andreas, and Jeanine P. Abrons.

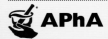
APhA

Medications with Adverse Withdrawal Effects from Abrupt Discontinuation – MODERATE to MILD

Medication Category	Medication Examples	Presentation with Abrupt Stop	Symptoms	Management/Risk Factors	Evidence	Potential to be Life Threatening
Nitrate	Isosorbide mononitrate & dinitrate (Imdur®, Isordil®)	Rebound angina	Mild to Severe	• **Management:** ○ Consider taper over 1 to 2 weeks use sublingual nitroglycerine as needed	Fair – Good	NO
Opioid	Oxycodone (OxyContin®) Hydrocodone (Hysingla®) Morphine (MS Contin®)	Flu-like symptoms; Insomnia; Anxiety; Cramps; Fatigue; Malaise	Mild to Severe	• **Management:** ○ Taper over 2 to 3 weeks if severe adverse effects, overdose, or with abuse. ○ Taper by ≤ 10% of original dose per week.	Good	NO
Antidepressant	Duloxetine (Cymbalta®) Paroxetine (Paxil®) Sertraline (Zoloft®) Venlafaxine (Effexor®) Desvenlafaxine (Pristiq®)	Flu-like symptoms; Insomnia; Nausea; Imbalance; Sensory disturbances; Hyper-arousal (FINISH)	Mild to Moderate	• **Risk factors:** ○ > 6 weeks use or short T½ • **Management:** ○ ↓ dose over weeks to months ○ Sub longer acting agent & ↓ every 2 to 3 weeks. ○ ↓ based on indication	Good	NO
Carbamate	Carisoprodol (Soma®)	Body aches; Sweats; Palpitations; Anxiety; Restlessness; Insomnia	Mild to Moderate	• **Management:** ○ Long taper: renal or liver impairment, age >65, TDD > 1400 mg, taper over 9 days* (specific taper schedule available) ○ Short taper: taper over 4 days*	Fair	NO

** *References Available Upon Request*

*** *List may not represent all medications, which have negative effects with abrupt discontinuation*

↑ **Classification of discontinuation symptoms & documentation based on the following criteria:**

- *Documentation: Excellent = package inserts, clinical trials, case reports/case series, reported & evaluated frequently in clinical literature; Good = package inserts, clinical trials, case reports/case series, reported & evaluated minimally in clinical literature; Fair = package inserts, case reports/case series, reported & evaluated minimally in clinical literature*
- *Discontinuation symptom severity: Severe = potentially life threatening with abrupt stopping; Moderate = bothersome, slightly less severe & non-life threatening symptoms; Mild = less severe symptoms but withdrawal reaction present*

Updated by Angela Wojtczak, Joanna Rusch, Elisha Andreas, and Jeanine P. Abrons.

Pharmacy Mnemonics

INTERACTIONS

Warfarin Interactions: <u>ACADEMIC FACS</u>

Amiodarone; **C**iprofloxacin/levofloxacin; **A**spirin; **D**icloxacillin; **E**rythromycin (macrolides); **M**etronidazole (azole antifungals); **I**ndomethacin; **C**lofibrates; **F**ibrates; **A**llopurinol; CYP 2C9 inducers/inhibitors; **S**tatins

CYP-450 Enzyme Inhibitors: <u>BIG FACES.COM</u>

Bupropion; **I**traconazole/ketoconazole/fluconazole; **G**emfibrozil; **F**luoxetine/fluvoxamine; **A**miodarone; **C**iprofloxacin; **E**rythromycin/clarithromycin; **S**ulfamethoxazole-trimethorprim; **C**lopidogrel; **O**meprazole/esomeprazole; **M**etronidazole

CYP-450 Enzyme Inducers: <u>PS PORCS</u>

Phenytoin; Smoking; **P**henobarbital; **O**xcarbazepine; **R**ifampin; **C**arbamazepine; **S**t. John's Wort

Simvastatin Increased Serum Levels: <u>ADIE</u>

Amiodarone; **D**iltiazem/verapamil; **I**traconazole; **E**rythromycin/clarithromycin

Prepared by Becky Petrik and Jeanine P. Abrons

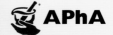

Pharmacy Mnemonics

SIDE EFFECTS

ACE Inhibitor: **CAPTOPRIL**

Cough; **A**ngioedema; **P**roteinuria/potassium excess; **T**aste changes; **O**rthostatic hypotension; **P**regnancy contraindication/pancreatitis; **R**enal failure/rash; **I**ndomethacin inhibition; **L**eukopenia/liver toxicity

Steroid: **BECLOMETHASONE**

Buffalo hump; **E**asy bruising; **C**ataracts; **L**arger appetite; **O**besity; **M**oonface; **E**motional changes (instability, euphoria); **T**hin arms and face; **H**yperglycemia/hypertension/hirsutism; **A**septic necrosis; **S**kin: striae, thinning, bruising (with topical preparations); **O**steoporosis; **N**egative nitrogen balance; **E**xtended wound healing

Morphine: **MORPHINES**

Miosis; **O**rthostatic hypotension; **R**espiratory depression; **P**neumonia; **H**istamine release/hormone changes; **I**nfrequency (constipation/urination); **N**ausea; **E**mesis; **S**edation

Increased Potassium (K$^+$) Levels: **K-BANK**

K$^+$ sparing diuretics/supplements; **B**eta blockers; **A**ngiotensin converting enzyme inhibitors (ACEI)/angiotensin receptor blockers (ARB); **N**onsteroidal anti-inflammatory drugs (NSAIDS); **K**idney disease

Prepared by Becky Petrik and Jeanine P. Abrons

Motivational Interviewing Techniques

Technique	Description	Example
Reframing/Rephrasing	• Strategy to help patients examine their perceptions in a different manner	• If a patient says people are always bothering me about quitting smoking – you could reframe to: Those people seem to care about you a lot.
Open-ended Questions	• Questions that a patient cannot answer yes or no to, but requires an explanation	• Questions which begin with who; what; when; where; how • What questions do you have?
Reflective Listening → Paraphrasing	• Listening carefully to your patients; really hearing what they are saying & allowing the patient to be the focus • Varying levels of depth may be used	• Statements can be used: You are not quite sure that you are ready to make a change, but you are aware that your current behavior may negatively impact your health or it's been tough
Re-stating	• Simply re-state what the patient has said	• Patient says "I'm frustrated." You say: "I understand, you are frustrated."
Readiness Ruler	• Scale from 1 to 7 • Asking patient how important the change is to them • First establish that it is of some importance (See example) • Next, establish that there is room for improvement (See example)	• Why a 3 & not a 1? • What would it take to move you from a 3 to a 7?
Modified Envelope Technique	• Helps the patient to identify their primary reason or focus for change	• If there was one thing that would motivate you to change, what would it be?

Prepared by Jeanine P. Abrons

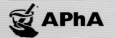

Pharmacists' Patient Care Process

Pharmacists' Patient Care Process

Pharmacists use a patient-centered approach in collaboration with other providers on the health care team to optimize patient health and medication outcomes.

Using principles of evidence-based practice, pharmacists:

Collect

The pharmacist assures the collection of the necessary subjective and objective information about the patient in order to understand the relevant medical/medication history and clinical status of the patient.

Assess

The pharmacist assesses the information collected and analyzes the clinical effects of the patient's therapy in the context of the patient's overall health goals in order to identify and prioritize problems and achieve optimal care.

Plan

The pharmacist develops an individualized patient-centered care plan, in collaboration with other health care professionals and the patient or caregiver that is evidence-based and cost-effective.

Implement

The pharmacist implements the care plan in collaboration with other health care professionals and the patient or caregiver.

Follow-up: Monitor and Evaluate

The pharmacist monitors and evaluates the effectiveness of the care plan and modifies the plan in collaboration with other health care professionals and the patient or caregiver as needed.

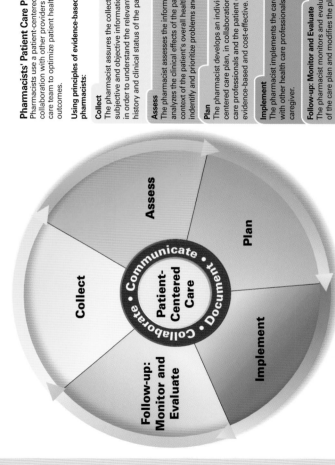

Source: Joint Commission of Pharmacy Practitioners, 2014